Copyright © 2020 by Anthony G. Puzzilla

All rights reserved.

No part of this publication may be reproduced, distributed or transmitted in any form or by any means, including photocopying, recording or other electronic or mechanical methods, without the prior written permission of the publisher, except in the case of brief quotations embodied in reviews and certain other non-commercial uses permitted by copyright law.

For permission requests please contact Canoe Tree Press.

Published 2020
Printed in the United States of America
Print ISBN: 978-1-7345504-0-5

Canoe Tree Press
4697 Main Street
Manchester, VT 05255
www.CanoeTreePress.com

Front Cover Illustration: As depicted by William R. McGrath, the *River Queen* (at the far left) would have hardly been noticeable among the throngs of cargo vessels in the teeming logistical center of City Point, Virginia, at the end of March 1865. (Hampton Roads Naval Museum Collection)

Contents

Dedication 7
Chapter 1 - Preface and Historical Setting 9
Chapter 2 - Railroads and Vessels as Strategic Targets 19
Chapter 3 - The U.S. Medical Department 27
Chapter 4 - The First Battle of Bull Run and its Aftermath 29
Chapter 5 - The Battle of Wilson's Creek 36
Chapter 6 - The Fort Henry and Fort Donelson Campaign 41
Chapter 7 - The Battle of Shiloh 45
Chapter 8 - The Harris Car 53
Chapter 9 - The United States Military Railroad 59
Chapter 10 - The Peninsula Campaign 63
Chapter 11 - The Battle of Seven Pines 79
Chapter 12 - The Battle of Savage's Station 84
Chapter 13 - Doctor Letterman 86
Chapter 14 - The Battle of Antietam 88
Chapter 15 - The Battle of Fredericksburg 95
Chapter 16 - The Chancellorsville Campaign 100
Chapter 17 - The Vicksburg Campaign 110
Chapter 18 - The Gettysburg Campaign 121
Chapter 19 - Battles of Fort Wagner 148
Chapter 20 - The Army of the Potomac 150
Chapter 21 - The Army of the Cumberland 160
Chapter 22 - The Battle of Chickamauga 169
Chapter 23 - The Battle of Chattanooga 172
Chapter 24 - The Battle of Trevilian Station 177
Chapter 25 - The Atlanta Campaign 180
Chapter 26 - The Battle of Nashville 193
Chapter 27 - The Campaign of the Carolinas 200
Chapter 28 - The South's Approach to Transporting its Wounded by Rail ... 206
Chapter 29 - Conclusion 210
About the Author 213

Contents

Dedication 7
Chapter 1 - Preface and Historical Setting 9
Chapter 2 - Railroads and Vessels as Strategic Targets 19
Chapter 3 - The U.S. Medical Department 27
Chapter 4 - The First Battle of Bull Run and its Aftermath 29
Chapter 5 - The Battle of Wilson's Creek 36
Chapter 6 - The Fort Henry and Fort Donelson Campaign 41
Chapter 7 - The Battle of Shiloh 45
Chapter 8 - The Harris Car 53
Chapter 9 - The United States Military Railroad 59
Chapter 10 - The Peninsula Campaign 63
Chapter 11 - The Battle of Seven Pines 79
Chapter 12 - The Battle of Savage's Station 84
Chapter 13 - Doctor Letterman 86
Chapter 14 - The Battle of Antietam 88
Chapter 15 - The Battle of Fredericksburg 95
Chapter 16 - The Chancellorsville Campaign 100
Chapter 17 - The Vicksburg Campaign 110
Chapter 18 - The Gettysburg Campaign 121
Chapter 19 - Battles of Fort Wagner 148
Chapter 20 - The Army of the Potomac 150
Chapter 21 - The Army of the Cumberland 160
Chapter 22 - The Battle of Chickamauga 169
Chapter 23 - The Battle of Chattanooga 172
Chapter 24 - The Battle of Trevilian Station 177
Chapter 25 - The Atlanta Campaign 180
Chapter 26 - The Battle of Nashville 193
Chapter 27 - The Campaign of the Carolinas 200
Chapter 28 - The South's Approach to Transporting its Wounded by Rail ... 206
Chapter 29 - Conclusion 210
About the Author 213

Copyright © 2020 by Anthony G. Puzzilla

All rights reserved.

No part of this publication may be reproduced, distributed or transmitted in any form or by any means, including photocopying, recording or other electronic or mechanical methods, without the prior written permission of the publisher, except in the case of brief quotations embodied in reviews and certain other non-commercial uses permitted by copyright law.

For permission requests please contact Canoe Tree Press.

Published 2020
Printed in the United States of America
Print ISBN: 978-1-7345504-0-5

Canoe Tree Press
4697 Main Street
Manchester, VT 05255
www.CanoeTreePress.com

Front Cover Illustration: As depicted by William R. McGrath, the *River Queen* (at the far left) would have hardly been noticeable among the throngs of cargo vessels in the teeming logistical center of City Point, Virginia, at the end of March 1865. (Hampton Roads Naval Museum Collection)

Acknowledgements

The author freely recognizes the scholarly contributions and works which have previously addressed, among other subjects, the role of railroads and hospital ships in the handling and transportation of wounded soldiers during the Civil War. These include:

Alan J. Hawk, National Museum of Health and Medicine, *An Ambulating History: or, How the Hospital Train Transformed Army Medicine* (September 2002) and *Hospital Ships in the American Civil War* (August 2005)

Robert R. Hodges, Jr., *American Civil War Railroad Tactics* (Osprey Publishing, August 18, 2009)

Frank R. Freemon, *Gangrene and Glory, Medical Care during the American Civil War* (University of Illinois Press, 2001)

Sanitary Commission, *Hospital Transports: A Memoir of the Embarkation of the Sick and Wounded from the Peninsula of Virginia during the Summer of 1862* (CreateSpace Independent Publishing Platform, December 24, 2012)

Anne L. Austin, "Nurses in American History: Wartime Volunteers: 1861-1865," *The American Journal of Nursing*, V. 75, no. 5 (May 1975)

Doctor L.P. Brockett and Mrs. Mary C, Vaughan, *Women's Work in the Civil War: A Record of Heroism, Patriotism and Patience* (Zeigler, McCurdy and Company, 1867)

John Vance Lauderdale, M.D., *The Wounded River* (Michigan State University Press, East Lansing, 1993)

George Washington Adams, *Doctors in Blue* (Louisiana State University Press, 1952).

Dedication

This book is dedicated to Terry Reimer, the Director of Research and the entire staff of the National Museum of Civil War Medicine located in Frederick, Maryland, in recognition of their dedication and commitment to telling the medical story of the Civil War—a story of care and healing, courage and devotion amidst the death and destruction of America's bloodiest war. This story is a tale of love and humanity displayed by unheralded men and women, of all color and persuasion, who unselfishly and heroically offered their compassion and care to both sides of this conflict. It is also a story of major advances, which occurred during these somber years which have had a lasting and profound impact on modern medicine.

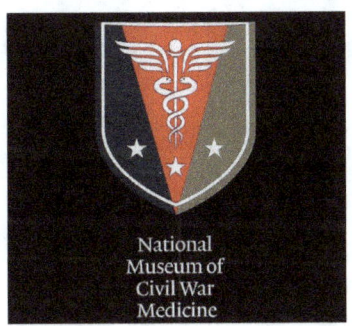

CHAPTER 1
Preface and Historical Setting

In 1861, when hostilities between the North and South formally erupted, our country had a rail network totaling more than 30,000 miles of track.

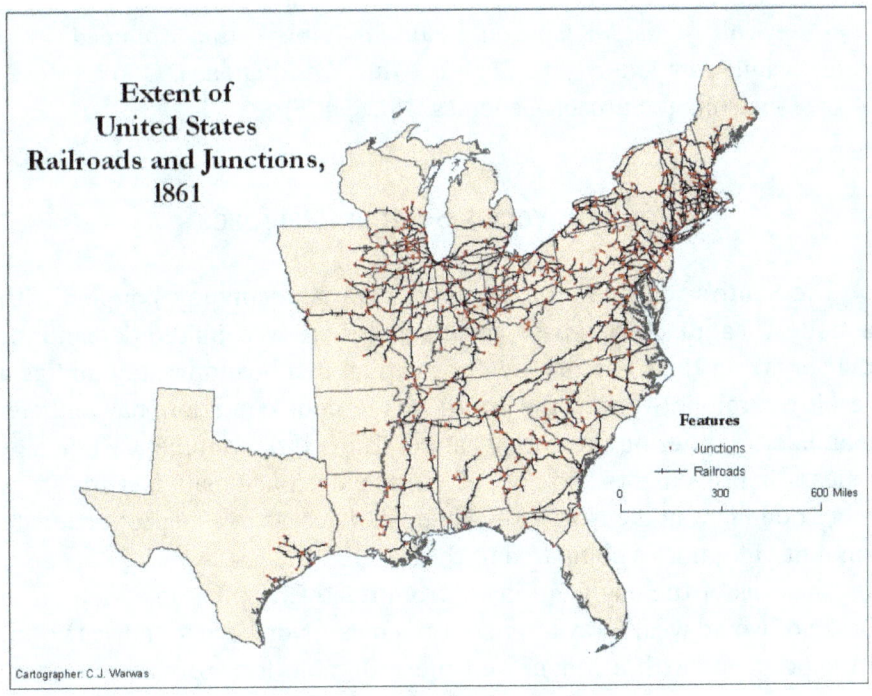

1-1: United States Railroad Lines, 1861

Of this, 21,300 miles or about 70 % was concentrated in the Northeast and Midwest while the Confederacy enjoyed only 9,022 miles of track. General McClellan wrote to Lincoln, "it cannot be ignored that the construction of railroads has introduced a new and very important element into war by the great facilities thus given for concentrating at particular positions large masses of troops from remote sections, and by creating new strategic points and lines of operations."

After the war, George Otis, the then Assistant Surgeon General wrote:

> "...The experience, discussions and experimental trials of various nations regarding railway transport of sick and wounded in war, indicates a very general solicitude for the determination of some regular system during the leisure time of peace. When the hour of need comes, imperious exigencies allow little opportunity for reflection and experiment on the means best adapted to meet the requirements ...and, unless provisions for their succor have matured beforehand, the comfort of the disabled must be sacrificed to inexorable military necessities."
> --George Otis, A Report on a Plan for Transporting Wounded Soldiers by Railway in Time of War (Washington, D.C., War Department, Surgeon General's Office, 1875).

Northern Versus Southern Railroads

The South's reliance on a primarily agrarian economy, coupled with a modest manufacturing base, meant that there was limited demand for rail service in the Confederacy. Less capital had been invested and as a result the rail network in the South was in poor condition, having been manufactured during the early years of railroad development when significant improvements had not yet been made. Since manufacturing was more dominant in the North, the Union had access to a disproportionate amount of foundries compared to the South.

The rails of the day were made from relatively soft iron which often broke or would wear away after continued use. Northern foundries began to experiment with stronger and more durable iron products such as steel. But the southern foundries had difficulty purchasing the necessary supplies for diligent upkeep of their rail lines, and as a result, the infrastructure of southern rail lines gradually crumbled. It has been estimated that during the Civil War, southern foundries could only manufacture 16,000 tons of railroad iron per year, yet 50,000 tons was required to adequately repair their deteriorating rail lines. To contrast that number, Pennsylvania foundries alone produced almost 270,000 tons of iron in 1860. Consequently even before war broke out, the South purchased most of their iron from Northern foundries. After the war began, the South outsourced, purchasing iron from Europe. However, the Union navy did their best to prevent this.

CHAPTER 1
Preface and Historical Setting

In 1861, when hostilities between the North and South formally erupted, our country had a rail network totaling more than 30,000 miles of track.

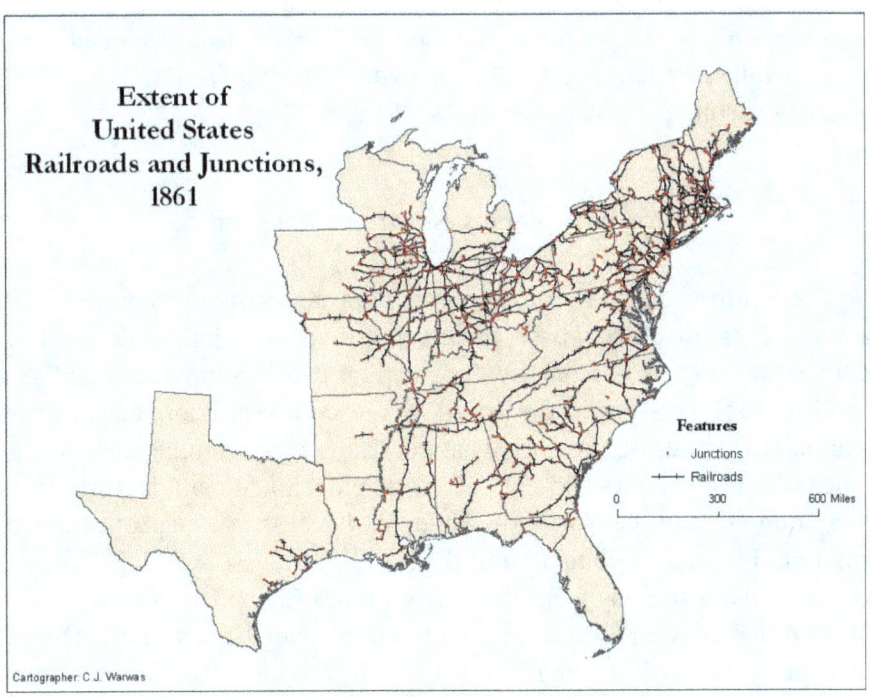

1-1: United States Railroad Lines, 1861

Of this, 21,300 miles or about 70 % was concentrated in the Northeast and Midwest while the Confederacy enjoyed only 9,022 miles of track. General McClellan wrote to Lincoln, "it cannot be ignored that the construction of railroads has introduced a new and very important element into war by the great facilities thus given for concentrating at particular positions large masses of troops from remote sections, and by creating new strategic points and lines of operations."

After the war, George Otis, the then Assistant Surgeon General wrote:

> "...The experience, discussions and experimental trials of various nations regarding railway transport of sick and wounded in war, indicates a very general solicitude for the determination of some regular system during the leisure time of peace. When the hour of need comes, imperious exigencies allow little opportunity for reflection and experiment on the means best adapted to meet the requirements ...and, unless provisions for their succor have matured beforehand, the comfort of the disabled must be sacrificed to inexorable military necessities."
> --George Otis, A Report on a Plan for Transporting Wounded Soldiers by Railway in Time of War (Washington, D.C., War Department, Surgeon General's Office, 1875).

Northern Versus Southern Railroads

The South's reliance on a primarily agrarian economy, coupled with a modest manufacturing base, meant that there was limited demand for rail service in the Confederacy. Less capital had been invested and as a result the rail network in the South was in poor condition, having been manufactured during the early years of railroad development when significant improvements had not yet been made. Since manufacturing was more dominant in the North, the Union had access to a disproportionate amount of foundries compared to the South.

The rails of the day were made from relatively soft iron which often broke or would wear away after continued use. Northern foundries began to experiment with stronger and more durable iron products such as steel. But the southern foundries had difficulty purchasing the necessary supplies for diligent upkeep of their rail lines, and as a result, the infrastructure of southern rail lines gradually crumbled. It has been estimated that during the Civil War, southern foundries could only manufacture 16,000 tons of railroad iron per year, yet 50,000 tons was required to adequately repair their deteriorating rail lines. To contrast that number, Pennsylvania foundries alone produced almost 270,000 tons of iron in 1860. Consequently even before war broke out, the South purchased most of their iron from Northern foundries. After the war began, the South outsourced, purchasing iron from Europe. However, the Union navy did their best to prevent this.

Southern rail lines also suffered from disconnect due to change in gauge, something that had happened as the rail networks evolved over time. North Carolina and Virginia shared the same type of gauge, standard gauge, yet the rest of the Confederate rail system operated on broad gauge. This disconnect kept much of the South isolated. Freight would have to be offloaded to another mode of transport, usually a wagon train, and then re-loaded onto another locomotive. Standardizing the gauge throughout the system during the war was not an option for the South, which lacked the time, money, and supplies to do this successfully. Once the North had captured a Southern rail line, it was effectively cut off from the rest of the network and rendered useless.

Even though the use of railroads, as a means of transporting passengers and commerce, pre-dated the Civil War, it was the very first time they played a major role in the conduct of a war. During the course of the war, railroads were second only to waterways in providing logistical support for both armies. Civil War railroad operations were characterized by the widespread use of locomotives and rolling stock to support armies tactically as well as logistically. They were used to move men, food, weapons and supplies to battlefield sites and encampments, including the evacuation of the wounded from these sites. The strategic map of the battles of the Civil War will be along the rail arteries of the country.

Medical evacuation trains were interchangeably known as hospital trains, ambulance trains, or sick trains. The use of so called "Hospital Trains" or "Ambulance Trains" actually originated during the Crimean War in the 1850s, but they weren't used in this country until the Civil War in both the North and South. These hospital trains had two basic functions: 1) transporting the sick and wounded to general hospitals in metropolitan areas either directly or to evacuation landings or ports where they would be then transported by vessel to these areas or 2) transporting the hospitals themselves or the so-called Mobile Hospitals or sometimes both of these functions.

The evolution and development of these hospital trains varied depending on the particular theater of war under consideration. Let's first consider the Western Theater of the American Civil War. Because of the generally longer rail travel distances involved between the actual battle sites and the location of the major metropolitan areas, and their general hospitals, the adoption and incorporation of new technological advances in the field of medicine, reflected in the design and operation of these hospital trains, was much more rapid and pronounced, especially in this theater.

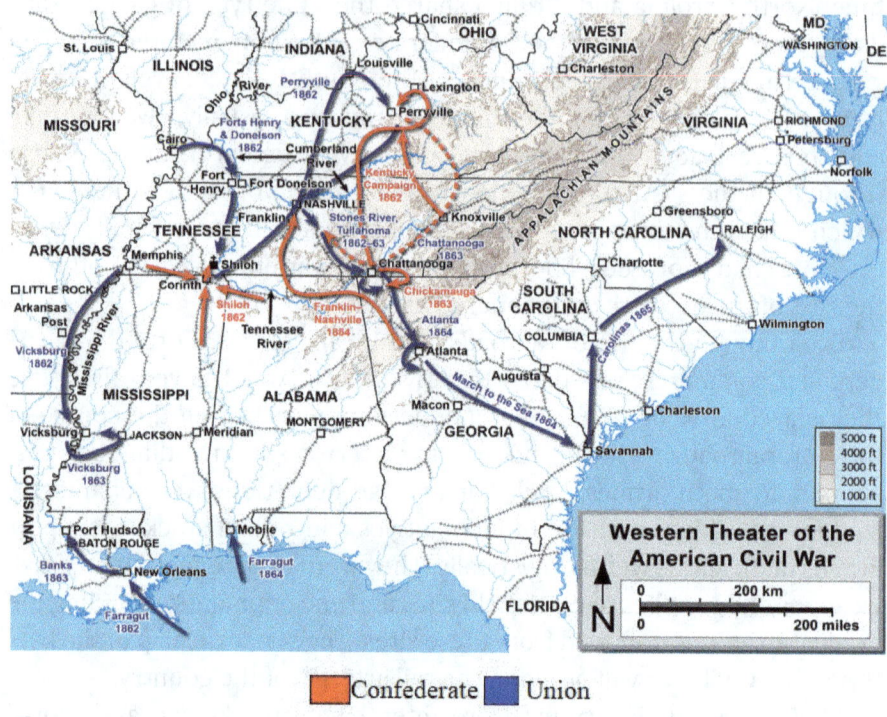

1-2: American Civil War Western Theater Overview

Therefore, in this theater, we see the development of sophisticated and advanced hospital rail cars supported, in the same train, by surgeon cars and fully equipped kitchens to care for and feed the wounded soldiers enroute to their ultimate destinations.

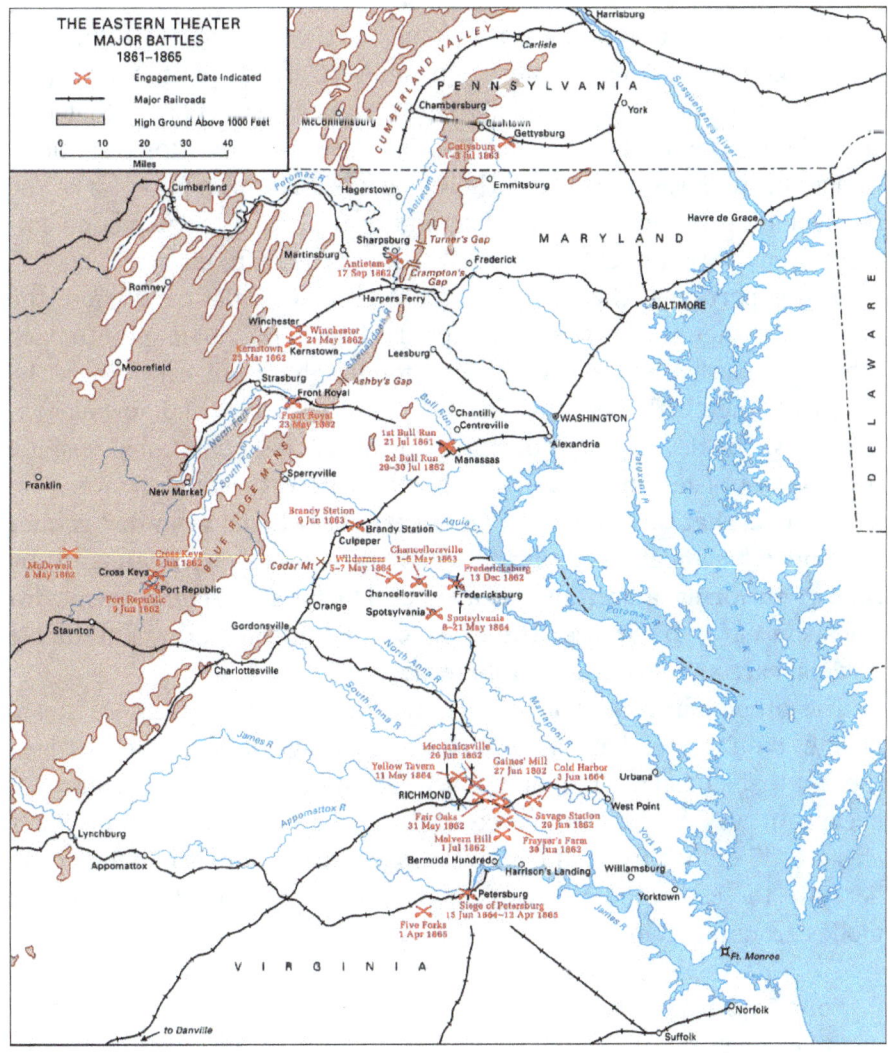

1-3: American Civil War Eastern Theater Overview

In contrast, in the Eastern Theatre of the American Civil War, many of the major battles like Antietam and Gettysburg saw the extensive use of dressing stations and field hospitals where the wounded were "medically stabilized" and then given emergency surgery, as necessary. Once they were sufficiently recovered from their wounds, they could be transported by rail to general hospitals in one of the many metropolitan areas are not far from the battlefield where they could receive long-term care. In addition, in Virginia where many of the battles of the Civil War were fought, the constant guerilla and cavalry raids on the railroad infrastructure encouraged the various Northern and Southern armies to use railroads in order to transport their wounded to the nearest dock or port so that they could be then moved by steamers to metropolitan areas for treatment. Hence, in the Eastern Theatre, there was a slower incorporation of the medical advancements for handling and transporting the wounded soldiers from the battlefields to general hospitals by railroad.

In this particular theater, we witness the use of flat cars where the wounded either climbed or were literally thrown on, holding on to each other for dear life, to the use of converted freight or box cars, where the floors are lined with hay, straw and/or blankets, being used now as hospital cars. The development of a fully contained and operational hospital train is not utilized, in the Eastern Theater, until very late in the war.

It seems that the longer the time between when a wounded soldier is deemed "medically stabilized," by his surgeon or physician, and the time of his formal admittance to a general hospital, and long-term convalescent care, the greater the need for sustainable and maintainable medical care and attention, while in transit.

The other major consideration is the fact that Civil War era steam engines didn't travel that fast, probably in the range of 15 to 20 mph. Given the fact that a hospital train probably traveled slower than a regular train, because it was carrying wounded soldiers, the top speed was probably closer to 15 mph. This sounds slow to us but to put things in perspective here are the estimated average speeds of contemporary transportation modes around that era:

Pony Express -- 7 to 10 mph
Stagecoach -- 3 to 5 mph
Horse & wagon (long distance) -- 2 to 4 mph (this was the preferred mode for the gold rush because it was so much faster than ox teams)
Ox team & wagon -- 1 to 2 mph (this was the preferred mode for most western pioneers as they could walk comfortably alongside the wagon and load more freight in the wagon)
Walking -- 2 to 3 mph
River boat (downstream) -- 5 to 10 mph
River boat (upstream) -- 1 to 5 mph

Prior to a battle, doctors established field dressing stations just out of range of enemy artillery. Once the battle was over, the wounded were considered to be non-combatants, in need of care, and nothing more. In theory, the wounded were carried from the battlefield by the Ambulance Corps, to a field dressing station in order to "stabilize" their wounds and then to the field hospitals for additional care, including surgery. Once cleared by the physicians and surgeons, as "healthy enough for travel," the wounded would then be transported by horse drawn ambulance and commissary wagons to a railroad depot where they would be sent directly to a general hospital in a metropolitan area or to a loading dock, pier or port where they were transported by vessel to metropolitan hospitals in Richmond, Lynchburg, Washington, Baltimore, Philadelphia and many other locations.

In the North, the sick and wounded were easiest and best removed by water, particularly in the vicinity of the Atlantic coast and in sections of the Mississippi watershed.

However, in the first months of the war, the medical evacuation of the wounded in the Union army by riverboat was at best totally absurd and ridiculous. The civilian captains of these vessels looked upon the sick and wounded as just another type of cargo; they refused to depart until the vessel was fully loaded, Very sick and wounded soldiers waited aboard without treatment and sometimes even without food until enough sick were available to fill the vessel. On other occasions, the sick and wounded were taken part of the way to the hospital center, but had to wait at an intermediate port while other cargo was handled. On the worst occasions, a line officer would insist that the ship, half loaded with wounded and half loaded with ammunition, must return to the battlefield to deliver the important cargo of ammunition. The sick and wounded were held at the intermediate port until other transportation became available or in the worst case.

This situation was further exasperated and reinforced by the charter of the Quartermaster's Department.

Before we proceed any further in our discussion, let's discuss briefly the Quartermaster's Department. This department was:

> "...charged with the duty of providing the means of transportation by land and water for all the troops and all the material of war. It furnishes the horses for artillery and cavalry, and for the

trains; supplies tents, camp and garrison equipage, forage, lumber, and all materials for camps; builds barracks, hospitals, wagons, ambulances; provides harness, except for artillery horses; builds or charters ships and steamers, docks and wharves; constructs or repairs roads, bridges, and railroads; clothes the army; and is charged generally with the payment of all expenses attending military operations which are not expressly assigned by law or regulation to some other department."

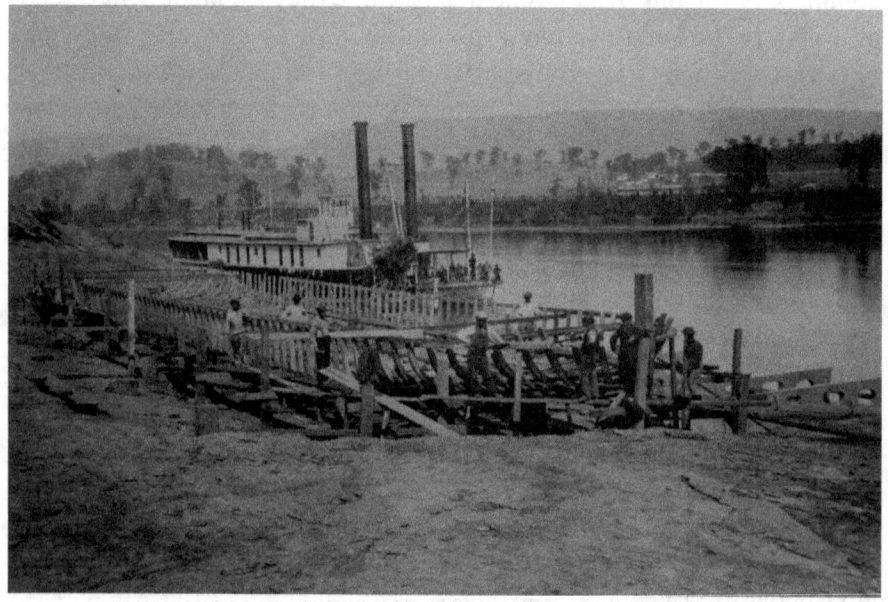

1-4: Men of the Quartermaster's Department building transport steamers on the Tennessee River at Chattanooga, 1864.

Hence, legislatively, at the beginning of the war, all transport vessels were under control of the Quartermaster's Department, which ordinarily gave the greatest preference and importance to its own duties. A surgeon needed request the Quartermaster's Corps to provide transportation for the sick these requests got low priority since the local quartermasters tended to put their efforts on the movement of troops, weapons, ammunition and supplies. In addition, the local quartermaster inundated by many transportation requests from colonels and generals often overlooked the request of the surgeon whose rank was equivalent to a major. As the efforts of the medical department were stymied, Medical Director

trains; supplies tents, camp and garrison equipage, forage, lumber, and all materials for camps; builds barracks, hospitals, wagons, ambulances; provides harness, except for artillery horses; builds or charters ships and steamers, docks and wharves; constructs or repairs roads, bridges, and railroads; clothes the army; and is charged generally with the payment of all expenses attending military operations which are not expressly assigned by law or regulation to some other department."

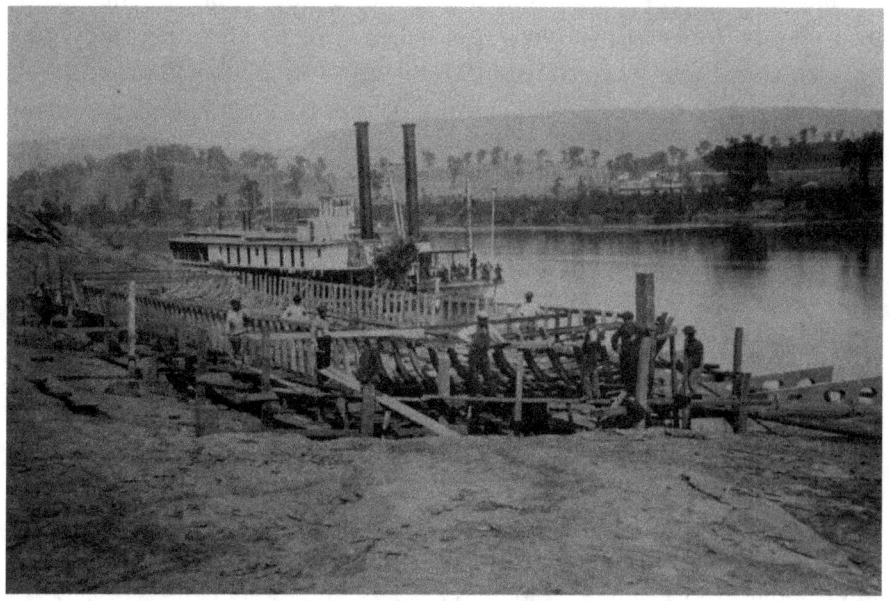

1-4: Men of the Quartermaster's Department building transport steamers on the Tennessee River at Chattanooga, 1864.

Hence, legislatively, at the beginning of the war, all transport vessels were under control of the Quartermaster's Department, which ordinarily gave the greatest preference and importance to its own duties. A surgeon needed request the Quartermaster's Corps to provide transportation for the sick these requests got low priority since the local quartermasters tended to put their efforts on the movement of troops, weapons, ammunition and supplies. In addition, the local quartermaster inundated by many transportation requests from colonels and generals often overlooked the request of the surgeon whose rank was equivalent to a major. As the efforts of the medical department were stymied, Medical Director

Prior to a battle, doctors established field dressing stations just out of range of enemy artillery. Once the battle was over, the wounded were considered to be non-combatants, in need of care, and nothing more. In theory, the wounded were carried from the battlefield by the Ambulance Corps, to a field dressing station in order to "stabilize" their wounds and then to the field hospitals for additional care, including surgery. Once cleared by the physicians and surgeons, as "healthy enough for travel," the wounded would then be transported by horse drawn ambulance and commissary wagons to a railroad depot where they would be sent directly to a general hospital in a metropolitan area or to a loading dock, pier or port where they were transported by vessel to metropolitan hospitals in Richmond, Lynchburg, Washington, Baltimore, Philadelphia and many other locations.

In the North, the sick and wounded were easiest and best removed by water, particularly in the vicinity of the Atlantic coast and in sections of the Mississippi watershed.

However, in the first months of the war, the medical evacuation of the wounded in the Union army by riverboat was at best totally absurd and ridiculous. The civilian captains of these vessels looked upon the sick and wounded as just another type of cargo; they refused to depart until the vessel was fully loaded, Very sick and wounded soldiers waited aboard without treatment and sometimes even without food until enough sick were available to fill the vessel. On other occasions, the sick and wounded were taken part of the way to the hospital center, but had to wait at an intermediate port while other cargo was handled. On the worst occasions, a line officer would insist that the ship, half loaded with wounded and half loaded with ammunition, must return to the battlefield to deliver the important cargo of ammunition. The sick and wounded were held at the intermediate port until other transportation became available or in the worst case.

This situation was further exasperated and reinforced by the charter of the Quartermaster's Department.

Before we proceed any further in our discussion, let's discuss briefly the Quartermaster's Department. This department was:

> "...charged with the duty of providing the means of transportation by land and water for all the troops and all the material of war. It furnishes the horses for artillery and cavalry, and for the

J. Simons received approval from Major General Henry Halleck to charter steamboats dedicated to the movement of the sick and wounded. Assistant Surgeon Alfred Henry Hoff was made Superintendent of Medical Transportation on the Mississippi River under General U.S. Grant. In this capacity, he oversaw the procurement and operations of the hospital ships. During his time he modified and supervised the D.A. *January*, the first hospital ship owned and operated by the government instead of the U.S. Sanitary Commission or another chartered ship.

It was not by chance that the Union Army followed the Ohio and Mississippi Rivers and their tributaries. These rivers were military highways. And what roads they were – with the Tennessee and the Cumberland Rivers running for hundreds of miles through the central part of the Confederacy.

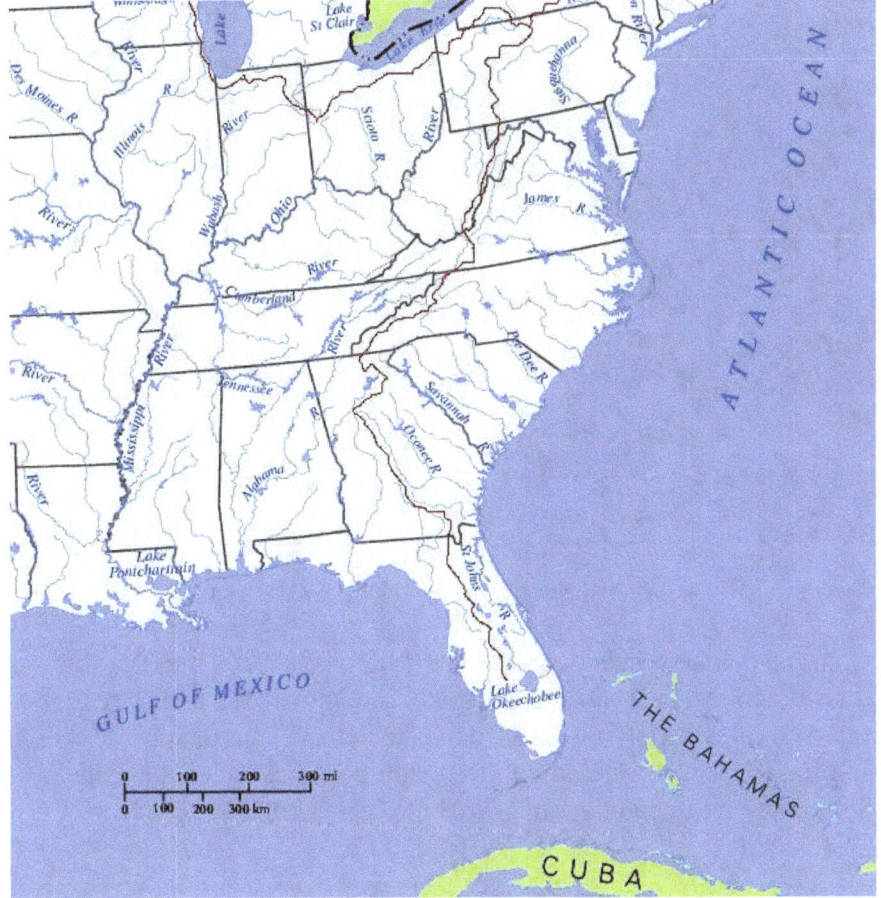

1-5 United States Rivers and Lakes

There are no known reports of the Confederate Army or Navy operating a dedicated hospital ship. The main reason for this is the fact that a Federal naval blockade (General Winfield Scott's Anaconda Plan) was instituted around all the principal Southern ports during the entire course of the war. In addition, the Confederates had planned to prevent penetration of their principal rivers with a series of well-defended forts, such as Fort Donelson on the Cumberland. Fort Henry on the Tennessee River, Island Number 10 on the upper Mississippi River and two forts below New Orleans. However the combined forces of the U.S. Navy and Army pushed past all these defensive positions in the spring of 1862.

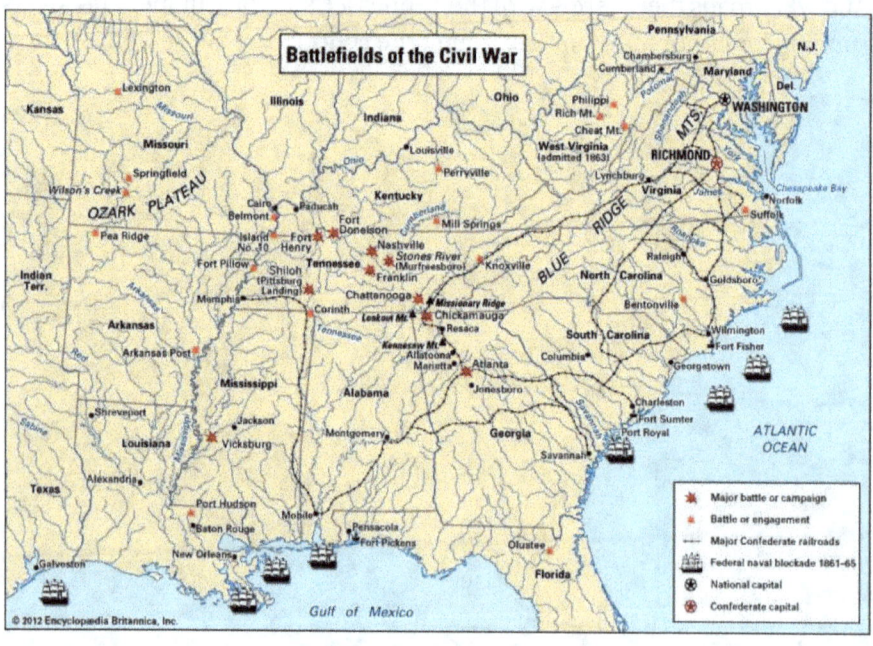

1-6: Battlefields of the Civil War

In general, the role of hospital ships in both theatres of the Civil War was transportation taking patients to medical care rather than as a place to provide medical care. Only the D.A. January, later renamed the Charles McDougall and the Red Rover were so outfitted with a surgical suite. Surgeons performed several amputations onboard both vessels while underway.

CHAPTER 2
Railroads and Vessels as Strategic Targets

The advantages of using railroads for shipping men and materiel to the front line quickly became obvious and railroad junctions became important strategic targets. Because of their strategic importance, railroads were frequently the target of attack, by opposing forces, which included railroad trains, railroad tracks, facilities, bridges, locomotives, rolling stock, and equipment.

A month before the First Battle of Manassas (July 21, 1861), Confederates ambushed an Alexandria, Loudon and Hampshire Railroad train loaded with Federal soldiers at Vienna, Virginia.

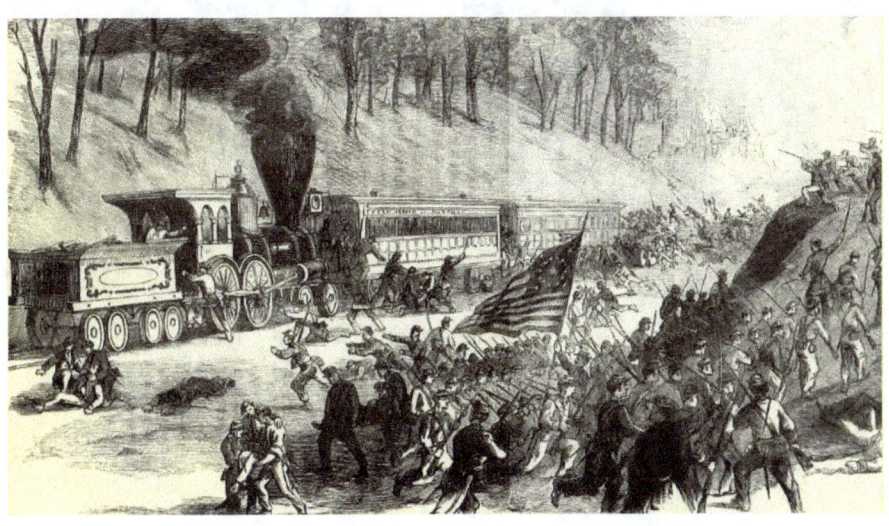

2-1: General Schenk, With Four Companies of the First Ohio Regiment, Surprised and Fired into by a Confederate Masked Battery near Vienna, VA June 17, 1861. Source: Frank Leslie's *Illustrated History of the Civil War*.

On Saturday afternoon, June 27, 1863, in scenic southern York County, Pennsylvania, Ticket agent Joseph Leib, Hanover Branch Railroad Conductor John Eckert, and their engineer and fireman are scrambling to get the steam up on their locomotive, the "Heidelberg," so they could escape oncoming Confederate cavalrymen, who were rapidly approaching Hanover Junction with an intent to destroy the railroad infrastructure and telegraph lines. Telegrapher Daniel Trone in Hanover had wired a warning, so Leib and company had plenty of foreknowledge the Rebels were coming.

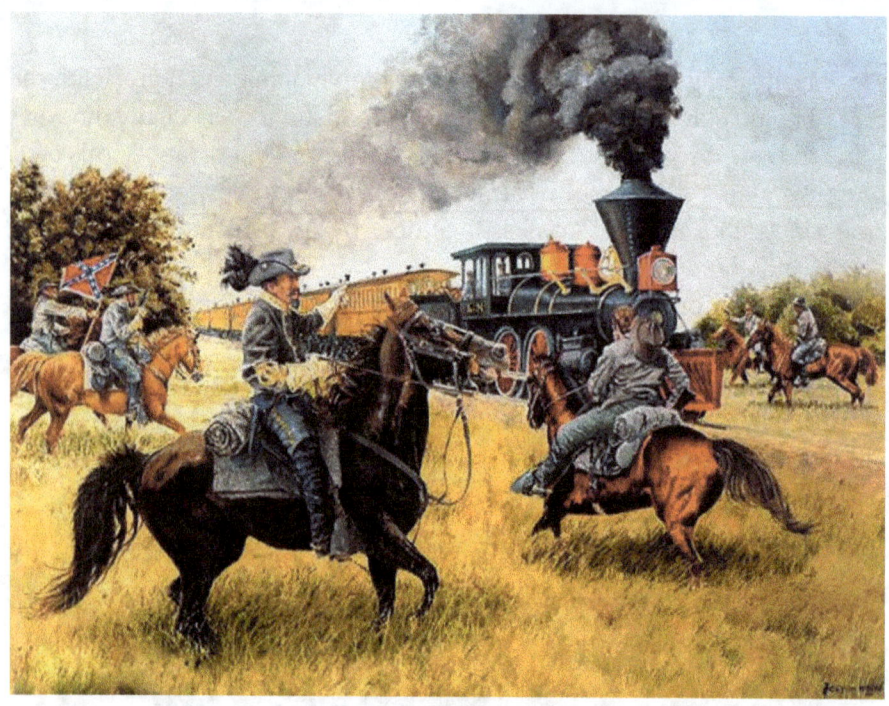

2-2: A way of sabotaging a locomotive that could not be saved by the enemy was to send it crashing off a bridge. This Federal ordnance train at Savage's Station in late June 1862 was set on fire and plunged into the Chickahominy River over what was left of Bottom's Bridge.

Railroads and Vessels as Strategic Targets | 21

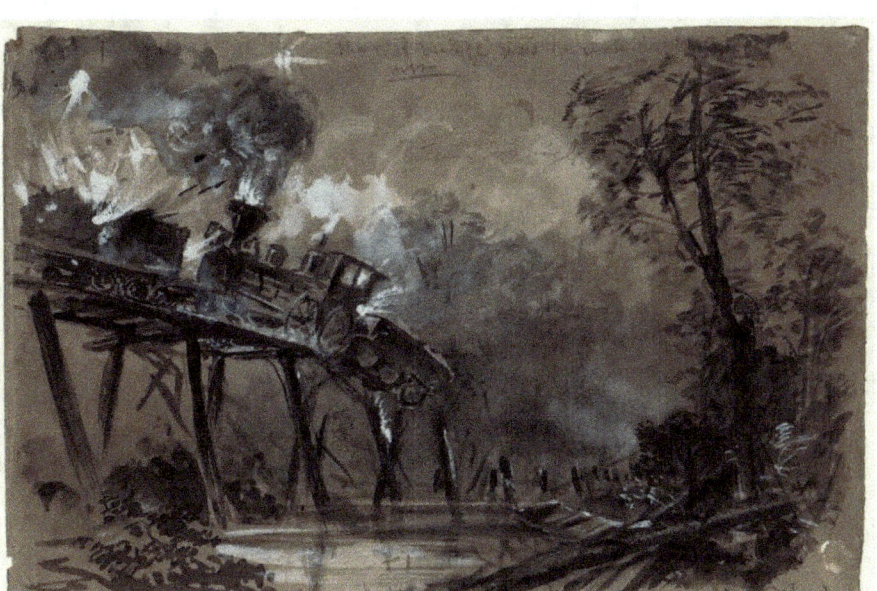

2-3: Confederate forces successfully derail a USMRR train as seen in this photograph during the war.

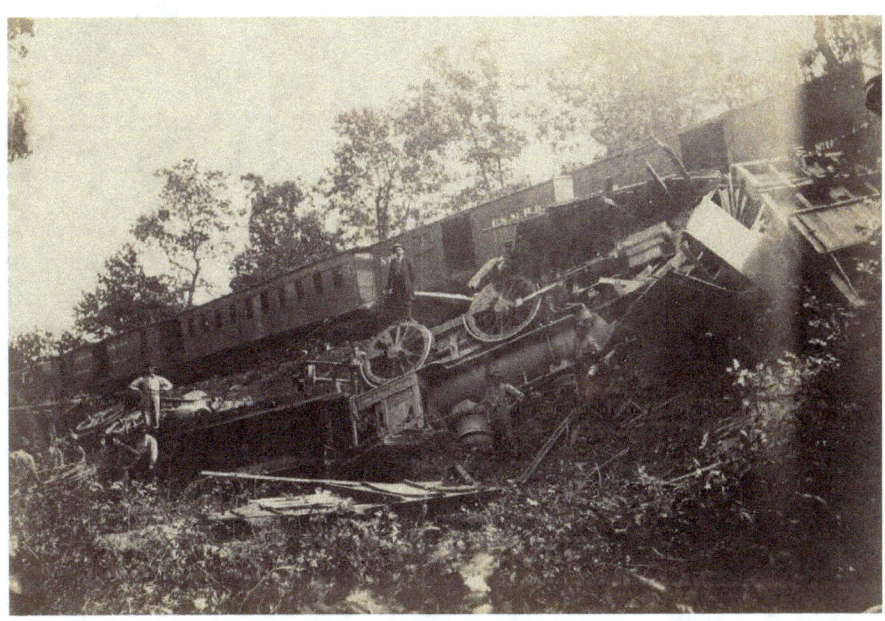

2-4: In 1862, Confederate forces celebrate the destruction of the critical Orange and Alexandria Railroad Bridge at Bull Run.

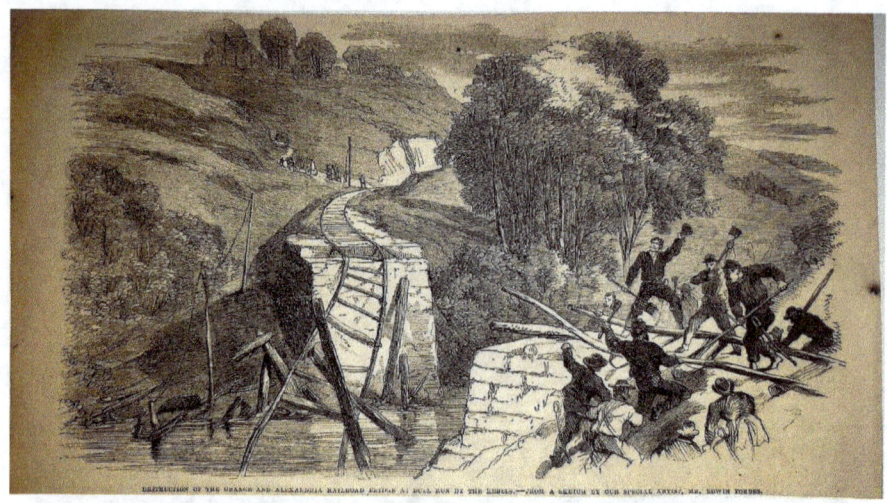

2-5: The Union forces raised havoc for the Confederacy by destroying the equally critical North Anna River Bridge, operated by the Richmond and Fredericksburg Railroad, in Virginia in May 1864.

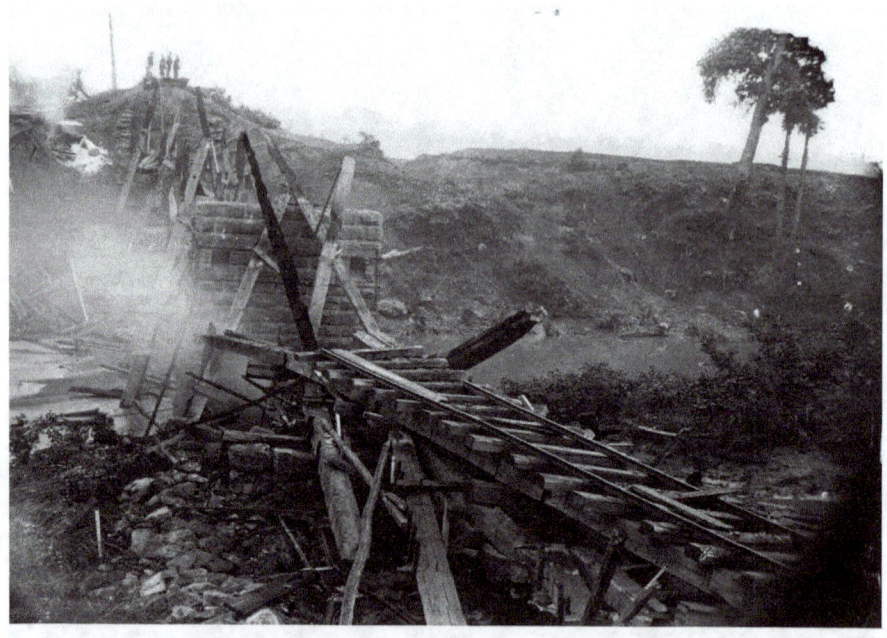

2-6: The deliberate burning of a wooden railroad bridge was sometimes necessary in order to impede the advancement of enemy forces.

For instance, in late June 1863, the Confederate Army had invaded Pennsylvania. After capturing York, the Rebels planned to take the state capital, Harrisburg, and possibly Philadelphia. To get there, they would need to cross the Susquehanna River at Wrightsville over the Pennsylvania Railroad rail line. Pennsylvania militiamen from Columbia, on the Lancaster County side of the river, vowed to block the Confederate advance. Union troops retreating from York joined them, as did a company of African American militiamen, the first Black troops from Camp William Penn. In all, they mustered fewer than 1,500 men. When Confederate Brigadier General John Brown Gordon arrived on June 28 with approximately 1,800 troops, the Federals were waiting in their entrenchments. The Rebels opened up with artillery fire, and the Union position rapidly became untenable. The Federals decided to retreat to Columbia and blow up a section of the over mile-long bridge behind them, denying the Rebels access to Lancaster. The explosion failed to destroy the bridge, so the order to burn it was given. As the Confederates surged forward, the bridge erupted in flames. Gordon's men worked for hours to extinguish the blaze. They kept Wrightsville from going up in smoke, but the bridge, financed by the First National Bank of Columbia, was destroyed. Gordon's brigade was recalled to York the next day. The Pennsylvania militia had saved Lancaster.

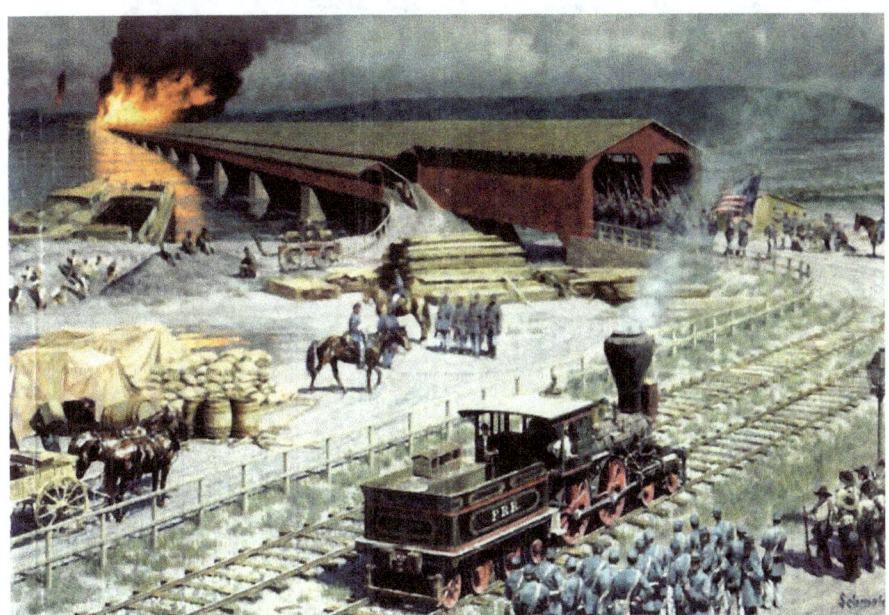

2-7: Burning of the bridge at Wrightsville.

24 | Hospital Trains and Vessels during the Civil War

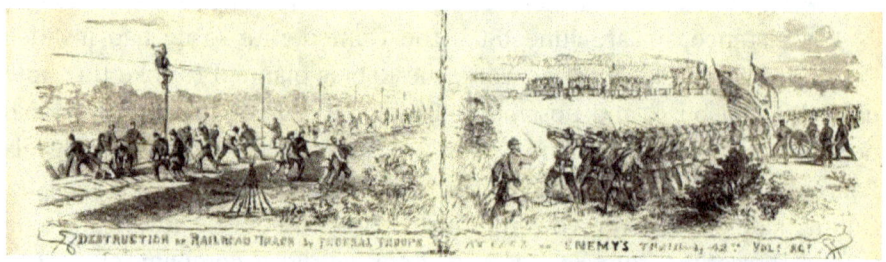

2-8: Frank Leslies's *Illustrated History of the Civil War* provided some interesting sketches showing the destruction of railroad tracks and an attack on a Confederate train by Federal troops.

Hospital ships on the James River were often fired upon and damaged from Confederate batteries placed on the banks near Harrison's Landing, just below Berkeley Landing, on the James River during the 1862 Peninsula Campaign.

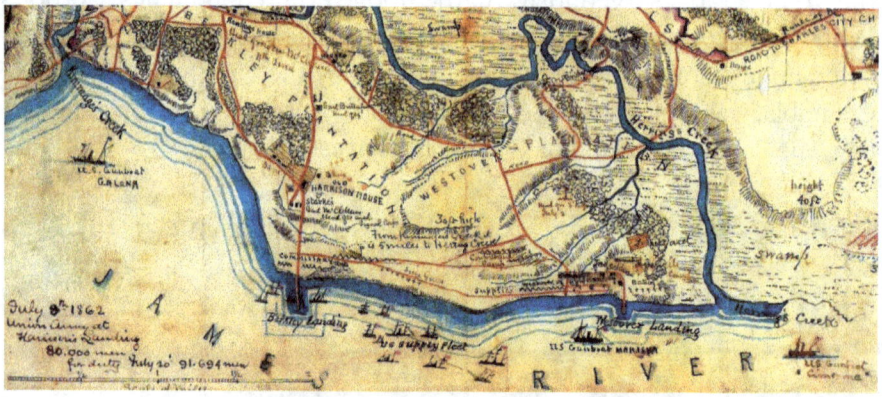

2-9: Map of the James River

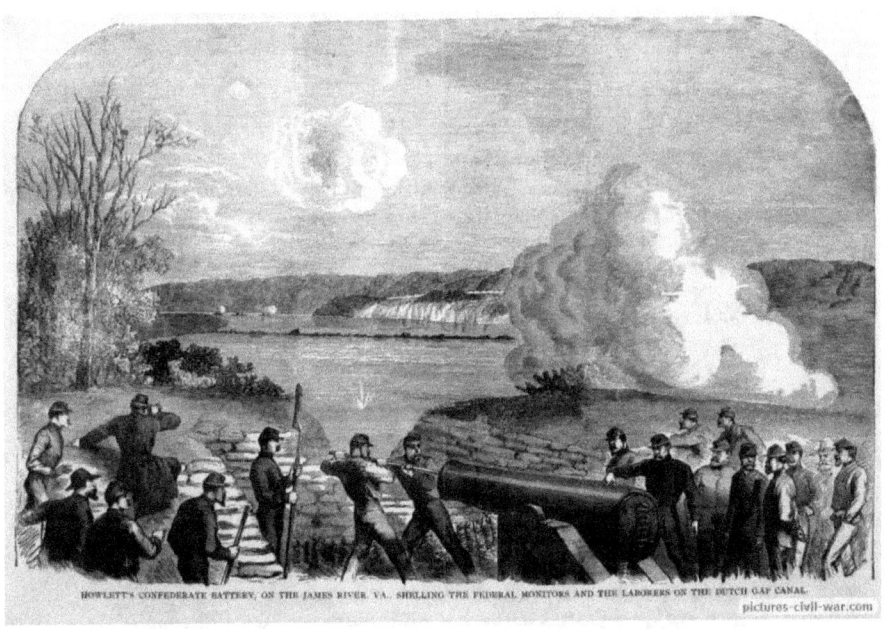

2-10: Battery at Dutch Gap on the James River

One such account involved the shelling of the hospital ship *Daniel Webster 2*, and other Federal steamers, as reported in the *Richmond Dispatch* of Thursday, July 15, 1862 at Harrison's Landing, Virginia:

Fights on the River—Movements of Burnside—Dispatches from McClellan, &c.

The Petersburg *Express*, of yesterday, has the following interesting news:

ANNOYING THE ENEMY.

On Thursday last a Confederate battery of eight guns having been placed in a position on James river commanding the channel below Berkeley, opened a very effective fire on several transports, convoyed by two or three gunboats, as they were ascending the stream. The river was narrow, and as the shot from our guns fell thick and fast among the Federal craft the consternation among the Yankees was great. The gunboats attempted to return the fire, but the elevated position of our guns rendered the enemy's fire comparatively harmless.

Over fifty shots were fired, striking several of the Federal craft and damaging them severely.—The large transport Daniel Webster crowded with troops, suffered more than any other—she, from some cause unknown to us, making slower progress in escaping from the scene of danger. In addition to the fire from our field pieces, we had some 250 sharpshooters lining the bank of the river, who poured repeated vollies on those occupying the decks of the steamers. Many must have been killed, the range being short and the sharpshooters comprising several of our most expert marksmen.

The Daniel Webster was lying but a short distance from Berkeley, Friday, apparently useless, many holes in her sides being distinctly visible, and her smokestack, railings, and other upper works, bearing palpable evidence of the damaging effects of the fire from our guns. Our men escaped without injury. The latter facts we learn from a gentleman who passed up James river Friday under a flag of truce from Old Point.

2-11: *Richmond Dispatch*, Thursday, July 15, 1862.

CHAPTER 3
The U.S. Medical Department

Let's pause for a minute to discuss the state of the U.S. Army Medical Department in 1861. At that time, the Medical Department did not have complete control over the care of the wounded. Evacuating the wounded to the rear was considered a logistical problem to be handled by the Quartermaster's Corps. While the Medical Department structure was adequate for the Mexican war and the small unit actions that followed, it could not handle the changing nature and sheer magnitude of warfare posed by the impending Civil War.

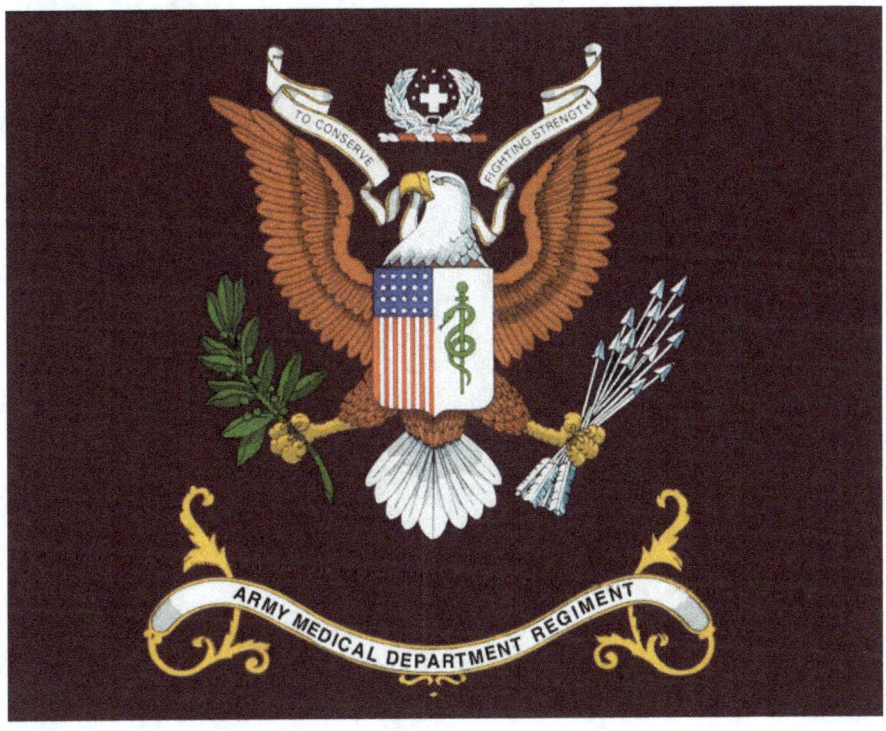

3-1: AMEDD Regimental Flag

In addition, one of the greatest challenges facing the Army Medical Department during the first three years of the Civil War was maintaining control over hospital ships. They did not have their own ships to transport wounded soldiers. Instead, they had to rely on ships borrowed from the U.S. Army Quartermaster's Corps that required refitting for medical uses. Furthermore, the U.S. Army Quartermaster's Corps frequently repossessed these vessels that they loaned to the Army Medical Department due to operational demands, stripping them of their medical transport configurations to allow for troop transport duty. When these vessels were finally returned to the Army Medical Department later, they would have to be refitted all over again, at enormous costs.

The Army Medical Department structure of 1861 would soon collide with the realities of combat in the First Battle of Bull Run.

CHAPTER 4
The First Battle of Bull Run and its Aftermath

The First Battle of Bull Run (the name designated by the Union), was referred to as the First Battle of Manassas by the Confederacy. The first battle of the Civil War was fought on July 21, 1861 in Prince William County, Virginia which is located just north of the city of Manassas and about 25 miles west-southwest of the city of Washington, D.C. Union forces totaling 28,450 were led on the field of battle by Brigadier General Irvin McDowell while Confederate Brigadier General P.G.T. Beauregard and General Joseph E. Johnston had 32,230 troops under their command. During the course of the battle, the Union suffered 1,124 wounded while the South had 1,582 wounded soldiers. The Union's forces were slow in positioning themselves which allowed Confederate reinforcements time to arrive by rail. The battle was considered to be a total Confederate victory which was followed by a disorganized rout of the Union forces back to Washington, D.C., along with a number of civilian onlookers.

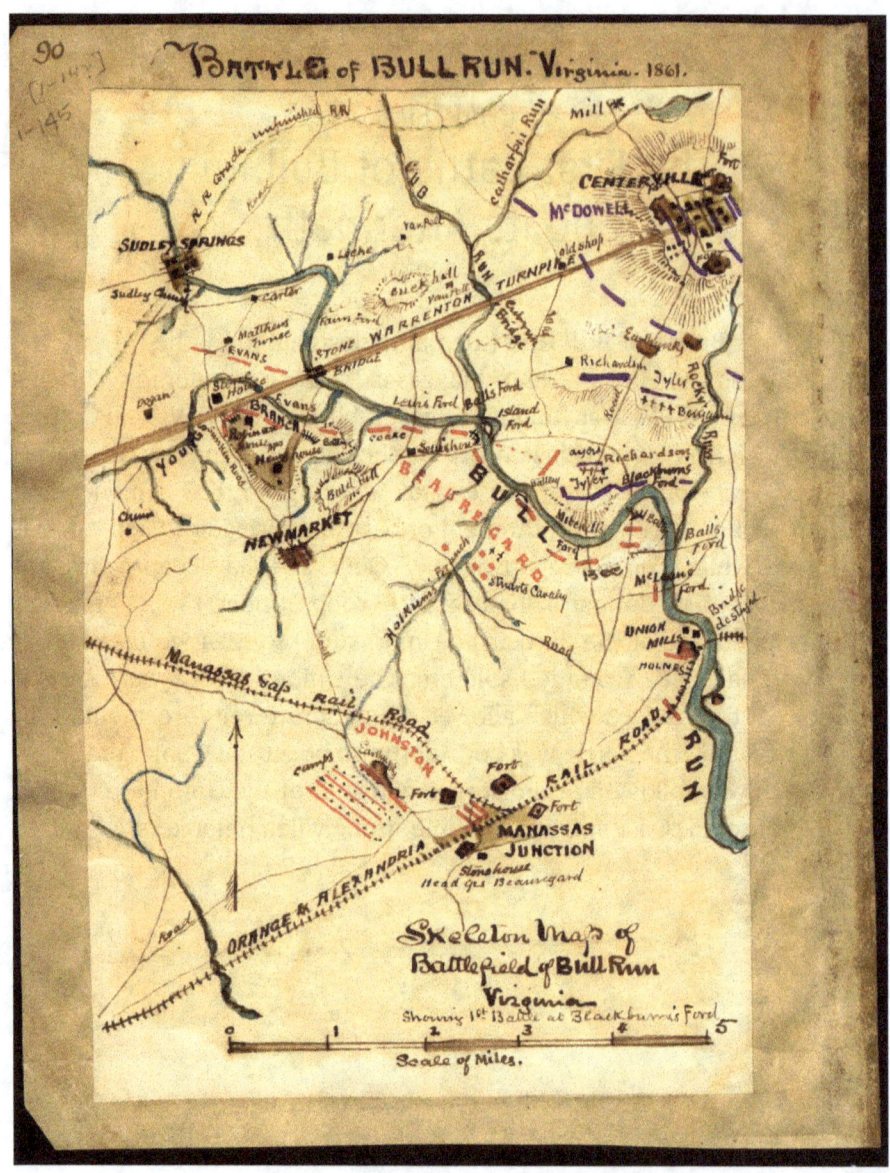

4-1: Map of the First Battle of Bull Run, July 21, 1861

The battle resulted in a complete rout of the U.S. Army forces as the retreating soldiers fled in panic back to Washington. The Union suffered 1,124 wounded as a result of the battle.

The Medical Department could not handle the sheer number of Union wounded. Regimental surgeons, since they worked for their unit only, were either swamped with casualties or were idle. Regimental band members and civilian ambulance drivers hired by the Quartermaster's Corps fled from the battle. Most of the wounded had to walk the 27-mile distance from the battlefield to Washington to reach the hospitals located there. Some of the more well-to-do Union soldiers actually checked into the Willard Hotel in D.C. and summoned their own physicians to tend to their wounds. Those wounded that couldn't make the walk remained on the battlefield for several days until they were picked up by ambulances, captured by Confederate forces or died from their wounds due to the lack of medical attention and care.

On the other side of the battle line, wounded Confederate soldiers were probably loaded onto converted freight cars, at Manassas Junction, most likely with little or no straw to soften their ride.

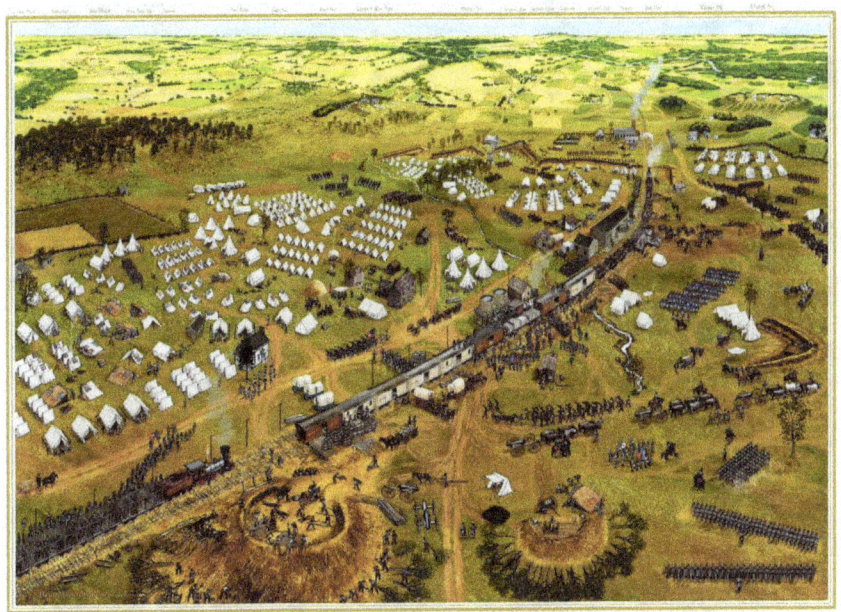

4-2: Manassas Junction, July 1861

These wounded Confederate soldiers then traveled to Charlottesville via the Orange and Alexandria Railroad sometimes also referred to as the Orange and Alexandria Railroad.

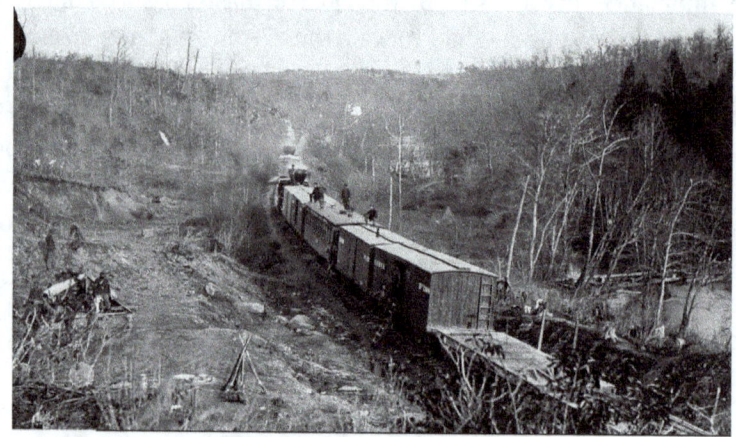

4-3: Orange & Alexandria Railroad

Still, getting to the General Hospital, in Charlottesville, Virginia could be a long, dangerous, and painful journey for many soldiers. It was twenty-four to thirty-six hours by train from Manassas Junction to Charlottesville, for instance, and at least one physician suggested that healthcare was not provided during the trip since they couldn't move between the cars while it was in transit.

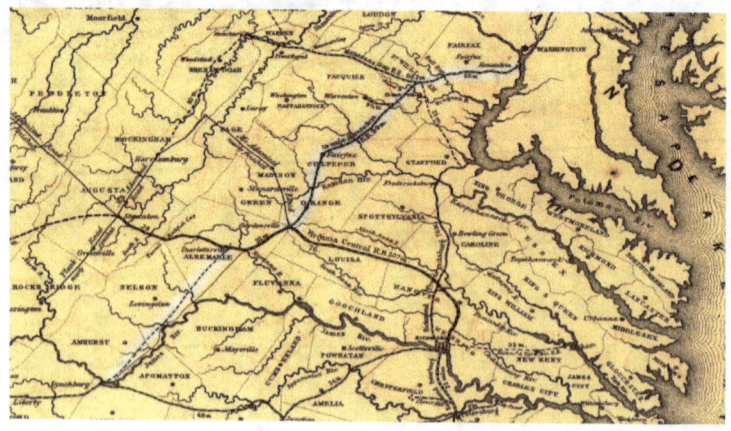

4-4: Orange & Alexandria Railroad Line

Opened in July 1861, the Charlottesville General Hospital began operations just in time to treat wounded soldiers from the First Battle of Bull Run, The need for general hospitals to serve the Confederate Army were needed and Charlottesville, Virginia was a logical location. Charlottesville was connected to Manassas Junction by railroad and made the transportation of wounded soldiers easier and would get them far enough outside the field of action.

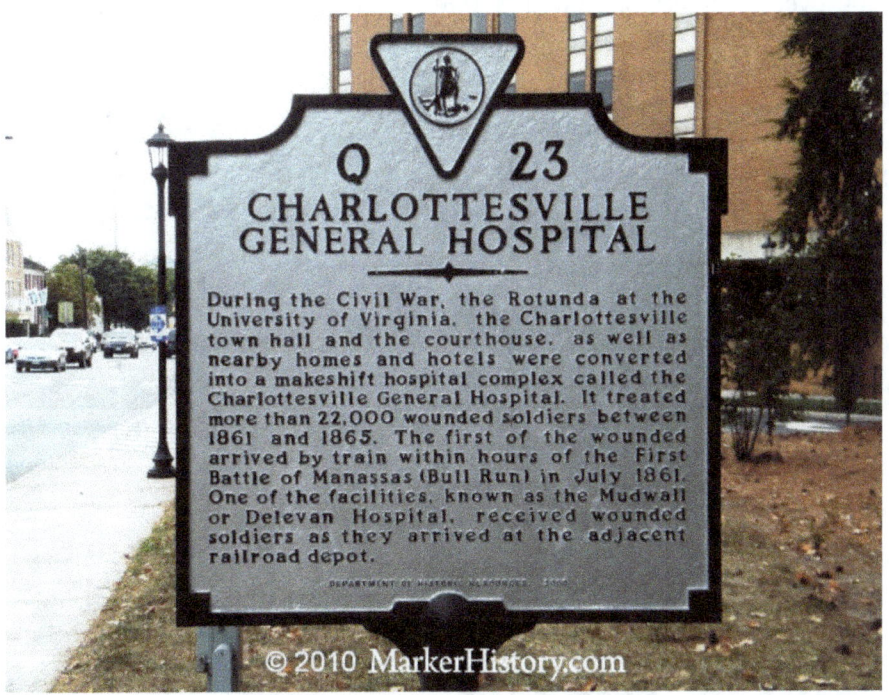

4-5: Charlottesville General Hospital

Outraged by the apparent incompetence of the Medical Department, following the First Battle of Bull Run, private citizens organized themselves in order to help take care of wounded soldiers. The most powerful of these organizations was the U.S. Sanitary Commission, which lobbied Congress and the War Department to reform the Army Medical Department. In addition to its political agenda, the Sanitary Commission funded hospitals, medical supplies and other facilities for wounded soldiers.

Volunteers from the Women's Central Association of Relief (WCAR) of New York witnessed the government's lack of sanitation and medical supplies. WCAR President Henry W. Bellows had traveled to Washington, D.C., intending to discuss matters regarding his organization. Meeting with Secretary of War Simon Cameron shortly after Bull Run, he instead discussed creating a Washington, D.C. organization that would provide advice and assistance to the Union military regarding medical care and general welfare. The War Department authorized the United States Sanitary Commission's on June 9, 1861, and President Abraham Lincoln approved its creation on June 13, 1861.

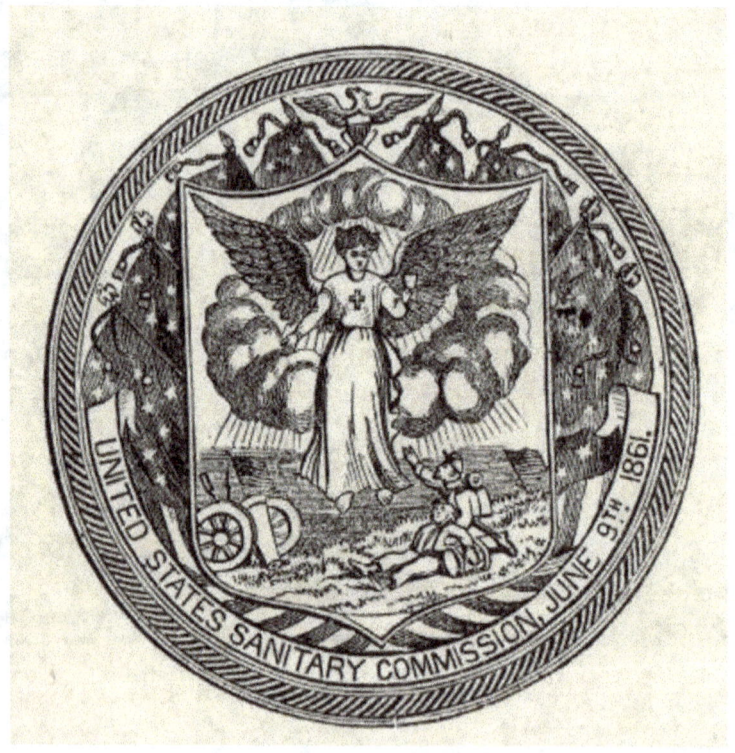

4-6: "Roughing It"

The U.S. Sanitary Commission, the only civilian-run organization recognized by the federal government, would serve as the focal point for civilian assistance to the military. U.S. Sanitary Commission volunteers advised on the physical and mental health of the military, assisted in the organization of military hospitals and camps, and aided in the transportation of the wounded by rail and by vessel. They conceived of the idea of hospital trains, supplied a number of hospital cars and operated the trains until the middle of the war when the military assumed responsibility for them. However, they continued to provide much of the medicine, food and other stores used in them. They distributed medical supplies, food, and clothing wherever needed. All of this was accomplished at no cost to the government, thanks to donations and their numerous fundraising activities.

Led by an executive board overseeing inspectors and field agents, U.S. Sanitary Commission branches in larger cities coordinated the efforts of local aid societies. Some existing regional aid societies, including the WCAR, would serve under the U.S. Sanitary Commission. Not everyone liked the idea of taking orders from Washington. Some organizations continued to function more or less independently, such as the U.S. Christian Commission which provided relief to both sides. On July 4, 1865, the U.S. Sanitary Commission ended its work. The last official act was the publication of its history in 1866.

CHAPTER 5
The Battle of Wilson's Creek

The Battle of Wilson's Creek was the first major battle in what was considered to be the Trans-Mississippi Theater of the Civil War. The battle was fought on August 10, 1861, near Springfield, Missouri. The state of Missouri was considered to be a neutral state even though its pro-South governor, Claiborne Fox Jackson, was actively collaborating with Confederate troops. In early August, Confederates under the command of Brigadier General Benjamin McCulloch and Missouri State Guard troops under Major General Sterling Price approached the forces of Brigadier General Nathaniel Lyon's Army of the West camped at Springfield. On August 10, Lyon, in two columns commanded by himself and Colonel Franz Sigel, attacked the Confederates on Wilson's Creek about 12 miles southwest of Springfield. Confederate cavalry were the first to be attacked and were forced to retreat from the high ground. Confederate infantry mounted three sustained attacks against the Union forces three times during the course of the day, but still failed to break their lines. When Lyon was mortally wounded and General Thomas William Sweeny was wounded, Major Samuel D. Sturgis assumed command of the Union forces. When Sturgis realized that his men were exhausted and lacked adequate ammunition to sustain the battle, he ordered a retreat to Springfield. The battle was deemed to be a Confederate victory, but the Confederates were too disorganized and ill-equipped to pursue the retreating Federal forces. Although the state stayed in the Union for the remainder of the war, the battle effectively gave the Confederates control of southwestern Missouri.

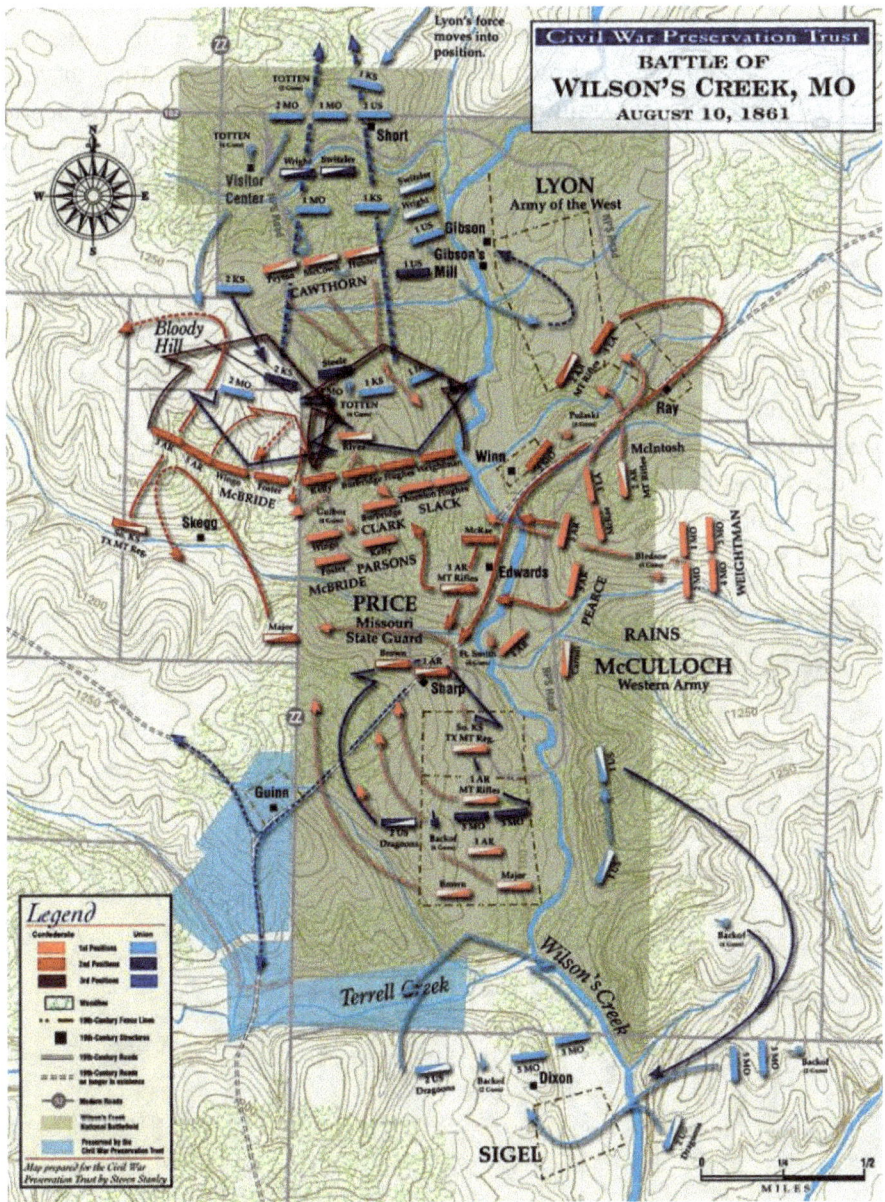

5-1: Wilson's Creek, Missouri

It is not clear who ordered the first medical evacuation by rail during the Civil War for the Northern Army which occurred after the Battle of Wilson's Creek on August 10, 1861. Medical preparations were inadequate since a Medical Director was never appointed for the effort. Hospital tents and ambulances were in short supply and the ambulance drivers had not received any training. Brigadier General Nathanial Lyons, leading the Missouri Volunteers, was killed in the battle and his troops were forced to retreat leaving 223 men killed and 721 wounded and 186 missing. Because of the shortages, the U.S. Army was forced to leave a number of its wounded soldiers, on the battlefield, to be captured by Confederate forces. The remaining wounded Union soldiers were placed under the care of Assistant Surgeon S. H. Melcher, Fifth Missouri Volunteers. He later reported to the Surgeon General on the evacuation of his patients: "I remained with two hundred and nine wounded and sick and, with the help obtained with convalescents they were made comfortable. During October, I sent one hundred and fifty of these patients to Rolla, (Missouri). On November 11th... I started with the remaining wounded, all of whom arrived safely in St. Louis on November 19th."

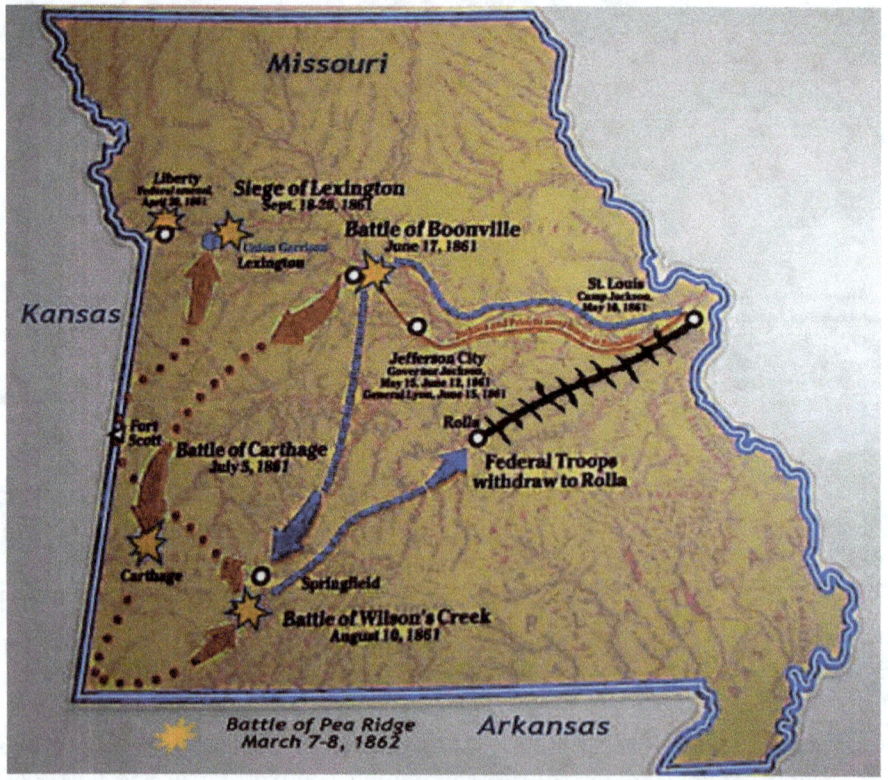

5-2: Theatre of Battle

Melcher did not mention the historic use of the railroad to move casualties in his report to the Surgeon General or discuss the efficacy of the hospital train. The report also understates how arduous a journey it must have been. Men recovering from gunshot wounds traveled over one hundred miles along a dirt road from the battlefield to Rolla, where they were loaded onto bare floors of boxcars and shipped an additional one-hundred and ten miles of unsettled railroad tracks of the Southwest Branch of the Pacific Railroad to the St. Louis City Hospital.

The jostling train ride was so painful that the soldiers improvised a system of placing tent poles in the sides of the boxcars and hanging stretchers with ropes from the poles. This system threatened to collapse with every creak of the railroad cars, frightening the wounded and their accompanying medical personnel.

As painful as the journey was to the wounded soldiers, it showed the potential of medical evacuation by rail to the Medical Department. It quickly became accepted practice because it made use of the empty railcars returning from the front and had minimal impact on the supply effort. The first hospital trains were improvised freight trains. Usually the floors of the boxcars were padded with straw, pine boughs and blankets. Some cars had the stretchers suspended from the ceiling by rope. "With this plan," wrote one surgeon, "a feeling of insecurity was common to the patients and attendants." A more stable arrangement used two or three tiers of litters that were securely lashed to a double row of upright stanchions.

While the trains did move the wounded to rear area hospitals quickly, the ride was excruciating. Soldiers, recovering from surgery or illness, had to endure the swaying, jarring and jolting of railcars with inadequate suspensions riding on uneven rails. Railcars, connected with link and pin couplings that which had up to six inches of slack, jammed together when the train stopped and jerked apart when the train started. Unless windows had been cut into the walls, ventilation was non-existent once the doors were closed for the journey. Katherine Wormeley, a Sanitary Commission official, described the conditions:

> "...the worst cases are put inside the covered cars, close, windowless boxes, sometimes with a little straw or a blanket to lie on, oftener without. They arrive a festering mass of dead and living together."

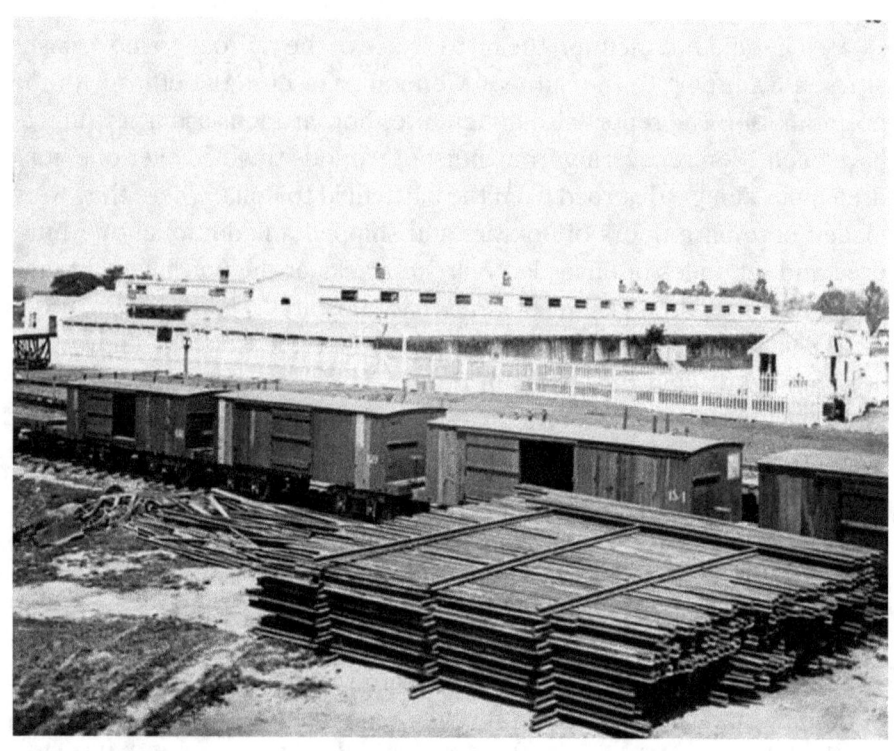

5-3: Civil War Boxcars

CHAPTER 6
The Fort Henry and Fort Donelson Campaign

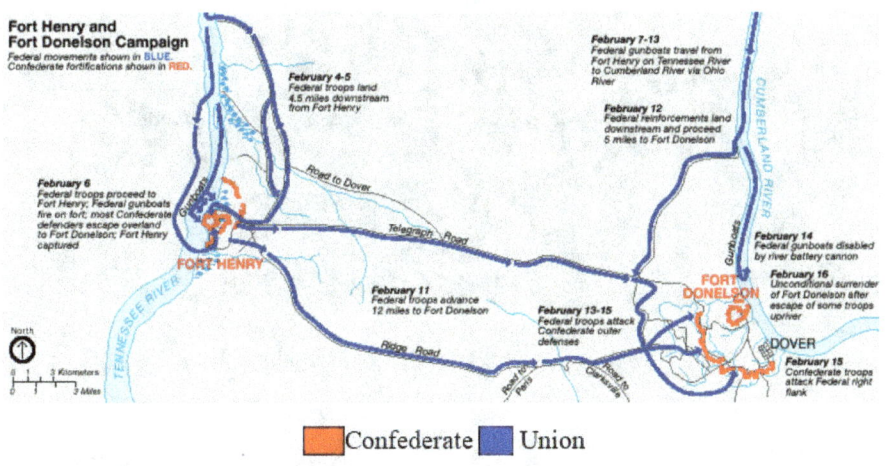

6-1: Fort Henry and Fort Donelson Campaign, February 6-16, 1862

To relieve the problem the sick and wounded being treated merely as cargo, riverboats were now dedicated to the transport of sick and wounded soldiers. The first vessel leased by military authorities for that purpose was the steamer *City of Memphis.* She had been refitted by the U.S. Sanitary Commission from a luxurious gambling river boat to a hospital ship capable of holding 750 beds. From February 7 to 18, 1862, she moored near Fort Henry on the Tennessee River. By March, she was joined by the steamboat *Louisiana.* The Western Sanitary Commission helped outfit that vessel by providing items not available to the Medical Purveyor. When completed, the *Louisiana* had four 100-bed hospital wards, each staffed by a medical officer, a ward master, six male nurses and one female nurse. In order to prevent passengers from joining the vessel, no one could be admitted on board as a patient without a written order by the Medical Director. Between February and July 1862, both the

City of Memphis and the *Louisiana* transported over 10,000 patients from ports in Tennessee to hospitals in Illinois, Ohio and Missouri.

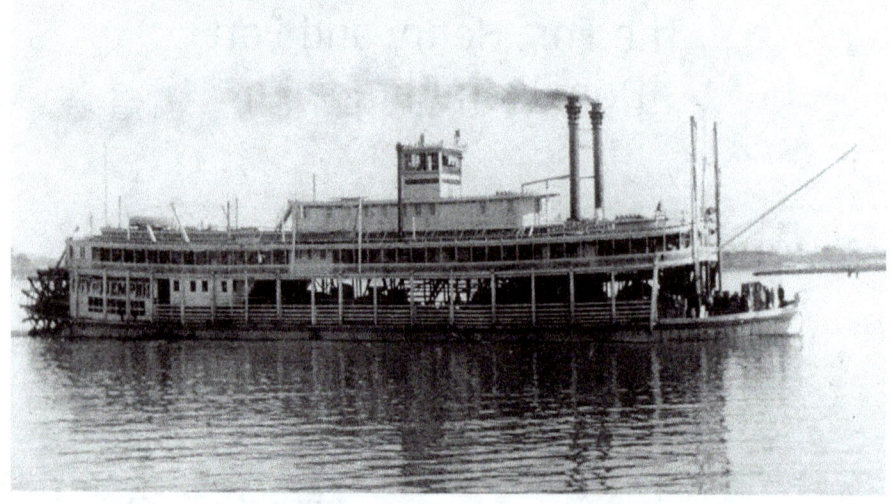

6-2: Hospital ship *City of Memphis*

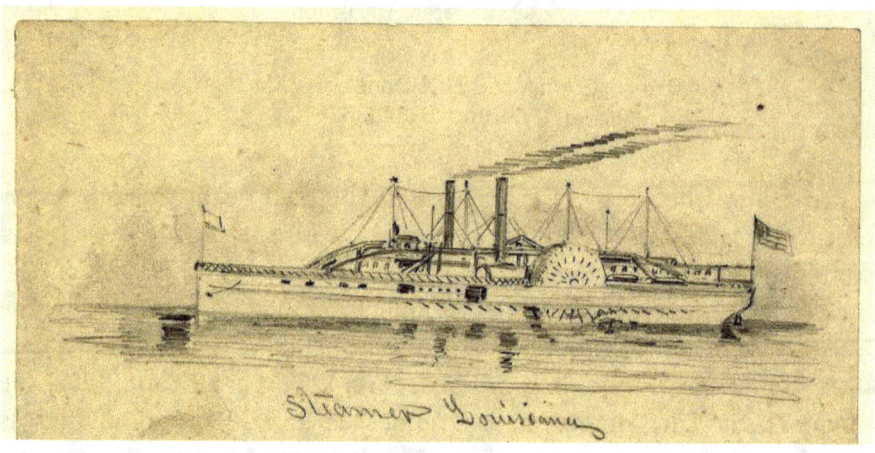

6-3: Hospital ship *Louisiana*

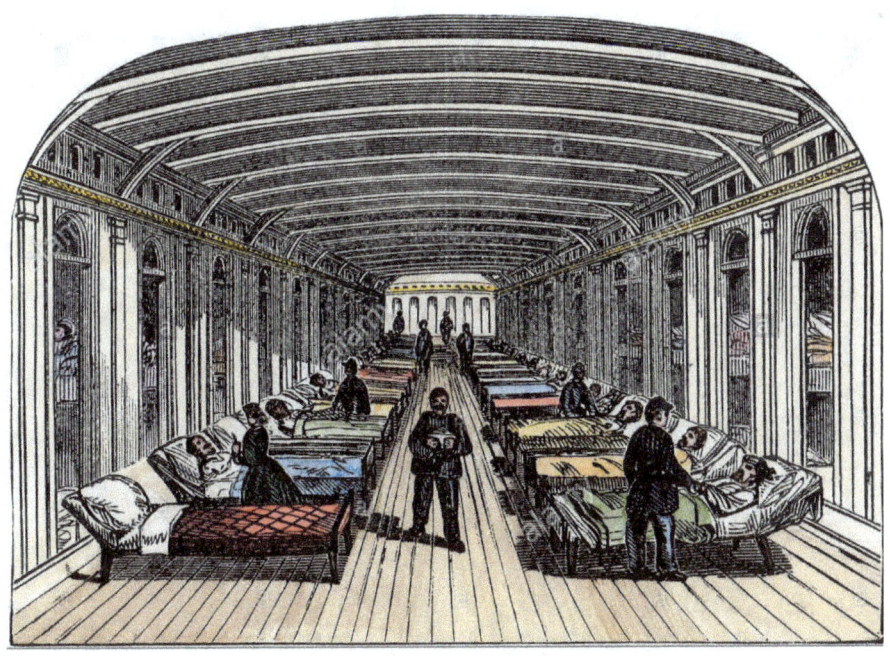

6-4: Interior of a typical steamer serving the Tennessee River during the Civil War.

Mary Ann ("Mother") Bickerdyke, a 44 year old widow with two young sons, began nursing Union troops at Cairo, Illinois in June 1861. After Mother Bickerdyke went to General Grant to plead for more adequate shelter for the wounded soldiers the Army commandeered a Cairo hotel and the General appointed her hospital matron. She stayed long enough to insure the hospital was meeting the soldiers' needs then left to nurse the wounded troops on the hospital ship *City of Memphis*.

44 | Hospital Trains and Vessels during the Civil War

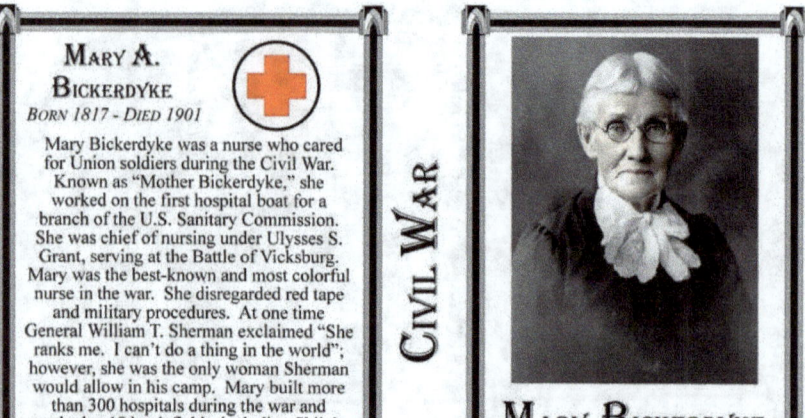

6-5: Mary Ann Bickerdyke (1817-1901)

CHAPTER 7
The Battle of Shiloh

The Battle of Shiloh, or as the Confederacy called it, the Battle of Pittsburg Landing, took place from April 6 to April 7, 1862. It was one of the earliest major engagements of the entire Civil War. The battle began when the Confederates launched a surprise attack on Union forces, known as the Army of the Tennessee, under leadership of Major General Ulysses S. Grant. He had moved his Union forces, via the Tennessee River, deep into Tennessee and was encamped principally at Pittsburg Landing on the west bank of the Tennessee River when the Confederate Army of Mississippi under Generals Albert Sidney Johnston and P. G. T. Beauregard launched their surprise attack. After initial successes, the Confederates were unable to sustain their positions and were forced back, which eventually resulted in a Union victory. Both sides suffered heavy losses, with more than 23,000 total casualties, and the level of violence shocked both the North and the South alike. The battle was the costliest in American history up to that point in time. The Union forces alone suffered 8,408 wounded while the South suffered 8,012 wounded during the course of the battle.

46 | Hospital Trains and Vessels during the Civil War

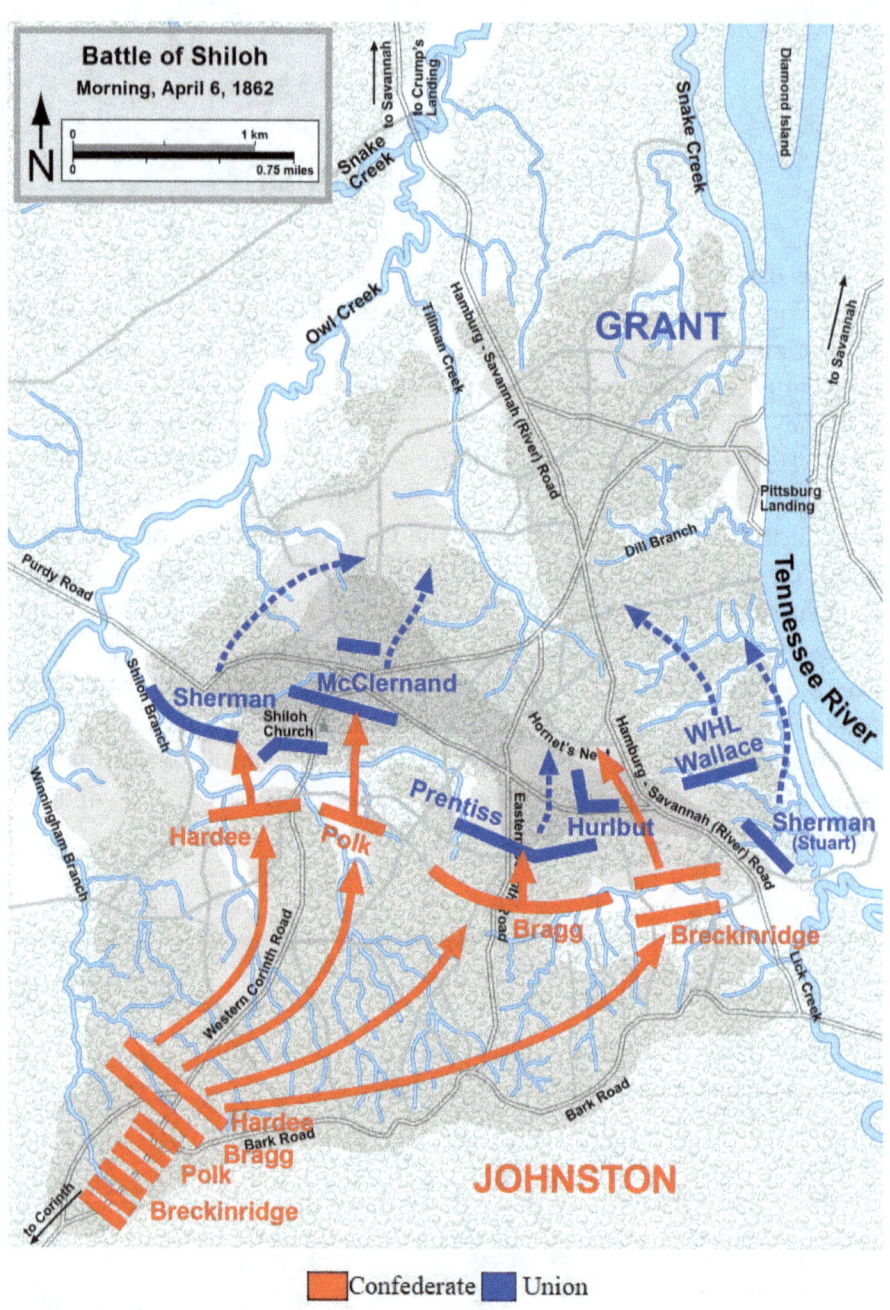

7-1: Battle of Shiloh

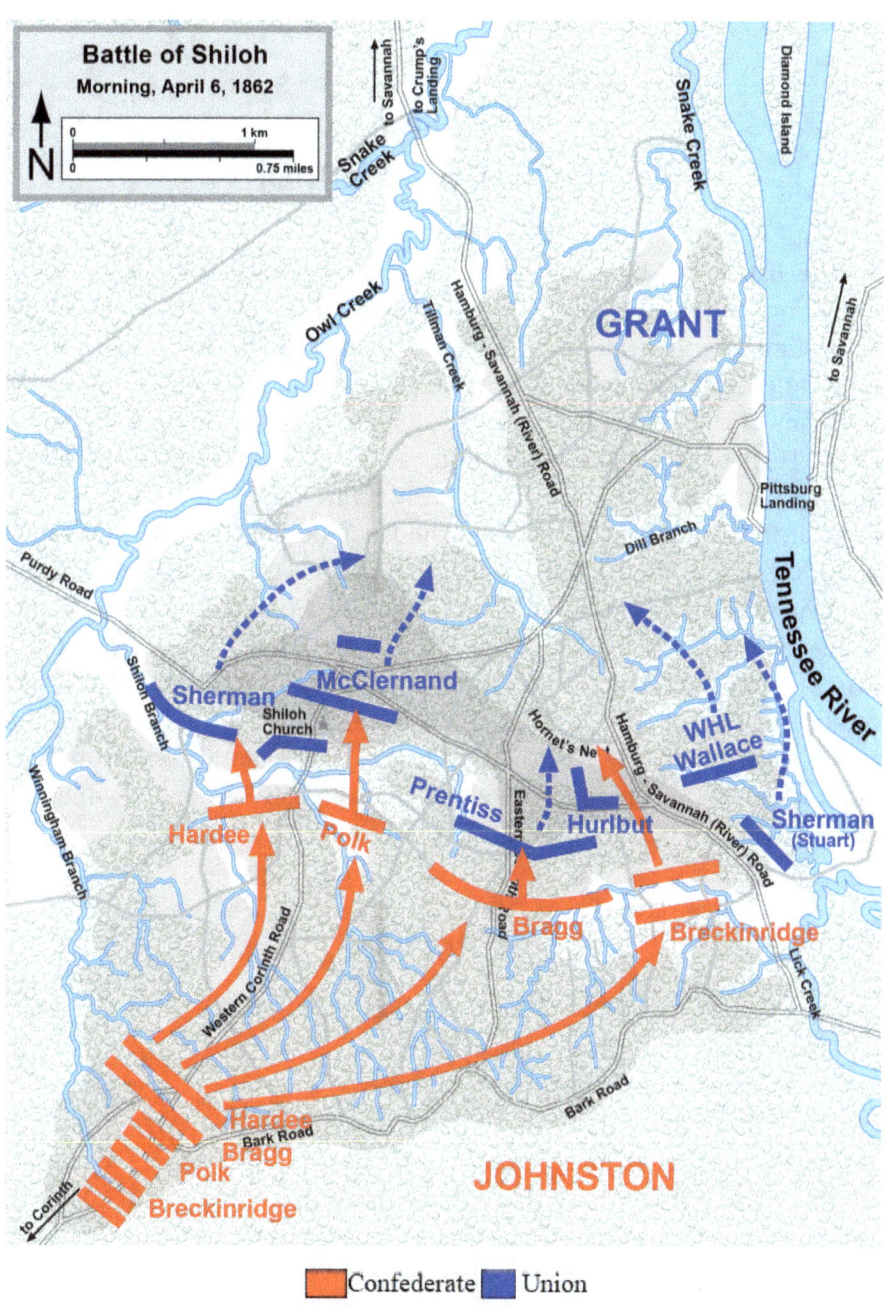

7-1: Battle of Shiloh

CHAPTER 7
The Battle of Shiloh

The Battle of Shiloh, or as the Confederacy called it, the Battle of Pittsburg Landing, took place from April 6 to April 7, 1862. It was one of the earliest major engagements of the entire Civil War. The battle began when the Confederates launched a surprise attack on Union forces, known as the Army of the Tennessee, under leadership of Major General Ulysses S. Grant. He had moved his Union forces, via the Tennessee River, deep into Tennessee and was encamped principally at Pittsburg Landing on the west bank of the Tennessee River when the Confederate Army of Mississippi under Generals Albert Sidney Johnston and P. G. T. Beauregard launched their surprise attack. After initial successes, the Confederates were unable to sustain their positions and were forced back, which eventually resulted in a Union victory. Both sides suffered heavy losses, with more than 23,000 total casualties, and the level of violence shocked both the North and the South alike. The battle was the costliest in American history up to that point in time. The Union forces alone suffered 8,408 wounded while the South suffered 8,012 wounded during the course of the battle.

Probably both Union and Confederate wounded were treated at one or more tent or canvassed field hospitals and, once medically stabilized by the surgeons, transported by ambulance wagons to Pittsburg Landing for transport by hospital ships. Pittsburg Landing a few days after the battle is the name of an engraving after an artwork by J.O. Davidson. It shows six transports at Pittsburg Landing shortly after the Battle of Shiloh, in April 1862. The one farthest up stream, on the right, is the *Tycoon* which was dispatched by the Cincinnati Branch of the U.S. Sanitary Commission with stores for the wounded. The next steamer is *Tigress* which was General Grant's headquarters boat during the Shiloh campaign. On the opposite side of the river is seen the gun-boat *U.S.S. Tyler*. The other known hospital ships, seen in this sketch of Pittsburgh Landing ships, were the other U.S. Sanitary Commission's transport *Monarch*, as well as the private and state hospital ships *Lancaster*, the *J.W. Hailman* and the *Marango*. Not appearing in this sketch was the D.A. *January* which transported wounded from Shiloh to St. Louis (431) and to Keokuk, Iowa (743). The vessel made a total of six trips to Pittsburgh Landing slowly dispersing an additional 959 wounded soldiers to hospitals along the Mississippi and Ohio Rivers from Cincinnati to Jefferson Barracks, near St. Louis.

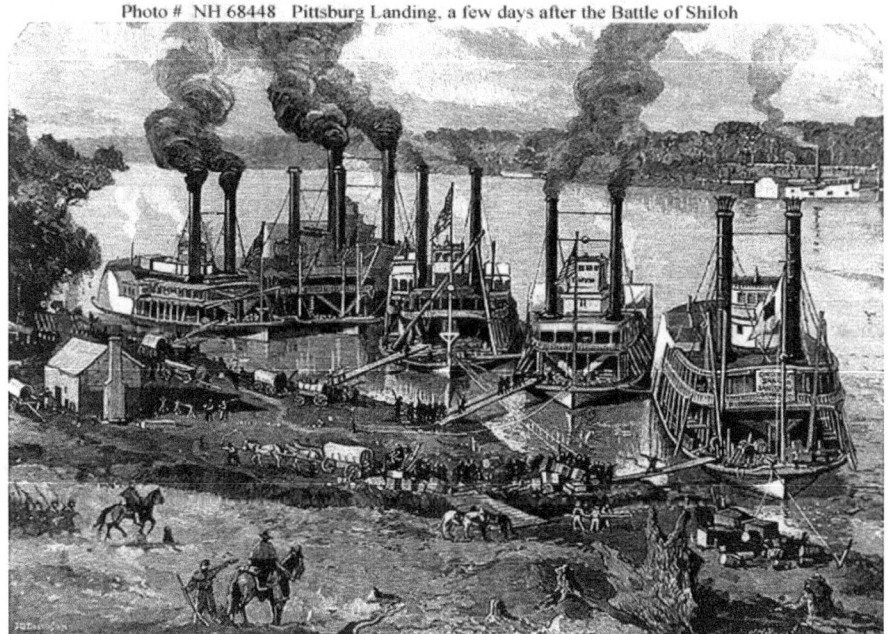

7-2: Riverboats at Pittsburgh Landing

Dr. John Vance Lauderdale related his experiences aboard the hospital ship D.A. *January* in his book *The Wounded River*. He fondly described the ship as follows:

> "For a hospital transport, the January was a tolerably handsome vessel, seaworthy in function and in appearance, which was certainly not true of some of the makeshift creations in the bizarre assortment of steamboats and ironclads that were rushed onto the river during the early days of the war."

In his book, he recorded his observations, following the Battle of Shiloh (April 6-7, 1862) aboard this steamer.

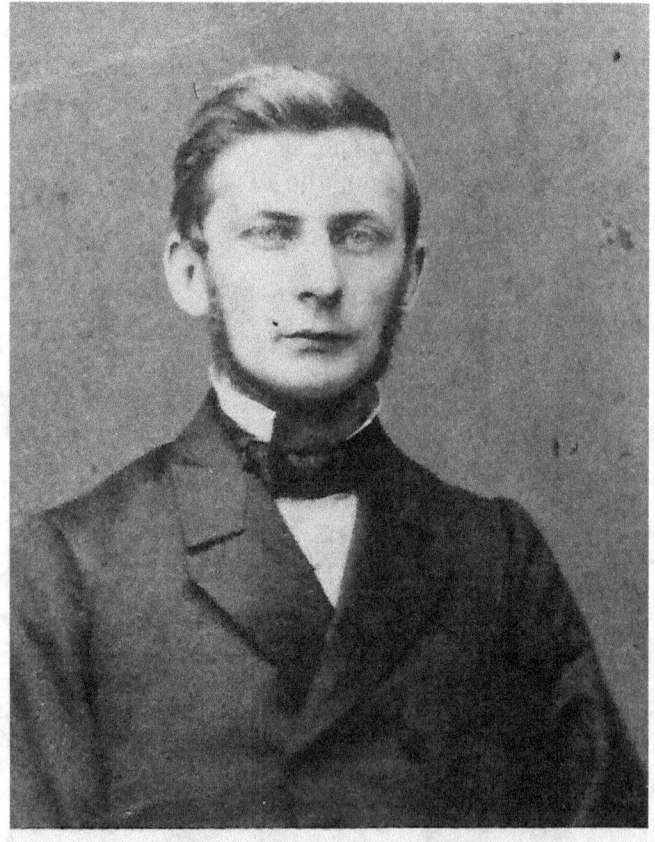

John Vance Lauderdale c. 1861

7-3: John Vance Lauderdale

In the following narrative of Dr. Lauderdale, the reference to Murray is Dr. Robert Murray is General Buell's medical director.

> "On the evening of April 7, one of Buell's surgeons, Dr. B.J.D. Irwin, imposed an ingenious order on the confusion by bringing together hundreds of infantry tents to construct the first recorded all-canvas field hospital, which he then artfully organized to shelter scores of patients from a cold, windswept hailstorm that pelted exposed wounds for three hours. As supply trains and hospital boats began to converge on the landing, a desperate plea for 10,000 mattresses went out over the telgraph. The call was answered with uncommon alacrity, but Murray lost no time waiting. After having the first of the ships 'fitted up with such bed-sacks as were on hand and with straw and hay for the wounded to lie upon, and filled to their utmost capacity,' he started evacuating the worst cases to general hospitals along the Ohio River."
> --The Wounded River, Dr. John V. Lauderdale

Miss Mary J. Safford, a native of New England, settled in Northern Illinois at the time of the Civil War.

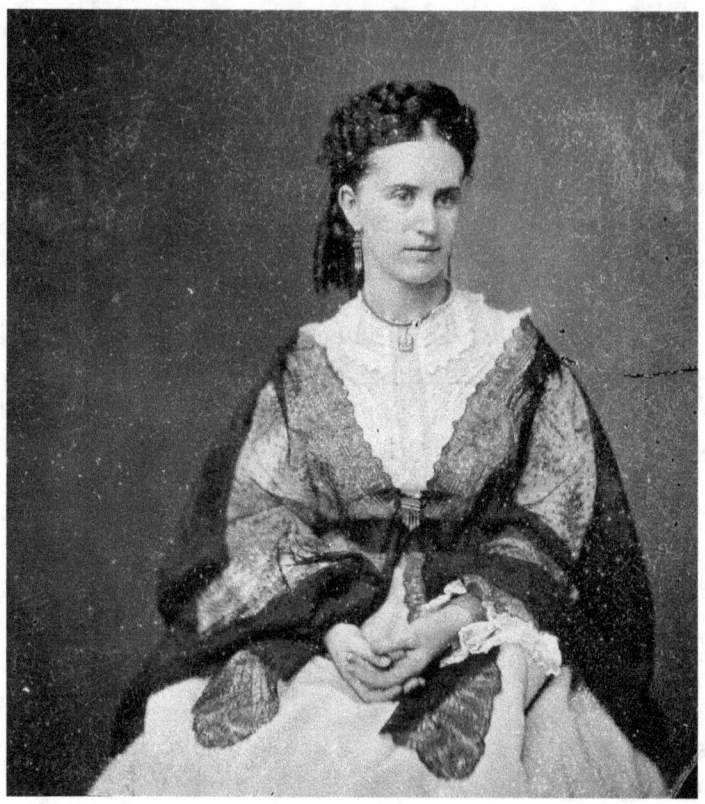

7-4: Mary J. Safford

She immediately became active in the war with the arrival of General Grant's soldiers in Cairo. Illinois. With the news of the Battle of Shiloh, she boarded a pair of military hospital ships on the Mississippi, the *City of Memphis* and the *Hazel Dell*, according to the book *Women's Work in the Civil War: A Record of Heroism, Patriotism and Patience*, written by L.P. Brockett and Mrs. Mary C. Vaughan:

> "As soon as the news of the terrible battle of Pittsburg Landing reached her, she gathered together a supply of lints and bandages, and provided herself with such stimulants and other supplies as might be required, not forgetting a good share of delicacies, and hastened to the scene of suffering and carnage, where she toiled incessantly day and night in her pilgrimage of love and mission of mercy for more than three weeks, and then

only returned with a steamboat-load of the wounded on their way to the general hospitals.

"At Pittsburg Landing, where she was found in advance of other women, she was hailed by dying soldiers, who did not know her name, but had seen her at Cairo, as the 'Cairo Angel.' She came up with boat-load after boat-load of sick and wounded soldiers who were taken to hospitals at Cairo, Paducah, St. Louis, etc., cooking all the while for them, dressing wounds, singing to them, and praying with them. She did not undress on the wayup from Pittsburg Landing, but worked incessantly."

The Confederate medical corps was simply overwhelmed by having over 8,000 badly injured casualties, at Shiloh, many of whom were mortally wounded. If one looks at a map of the railroads (below) in Mississippi one can see where the men were sent for medical care. The cities of Meridian and Tupelo were on the Ohio and Mobile Railroad right-of-way while Oxford was on the Mississippi Central Railroad route. Both railroads desperately sent the wounded Confederate soldiers to homes and schools at these locations that had not been near any combat and might have doctors and facilities available to care for the wounded. Since both of these railroads were predominantly freight carriers, one might assume that the handling and transportation of these wounded was rather crude and painful, at best.

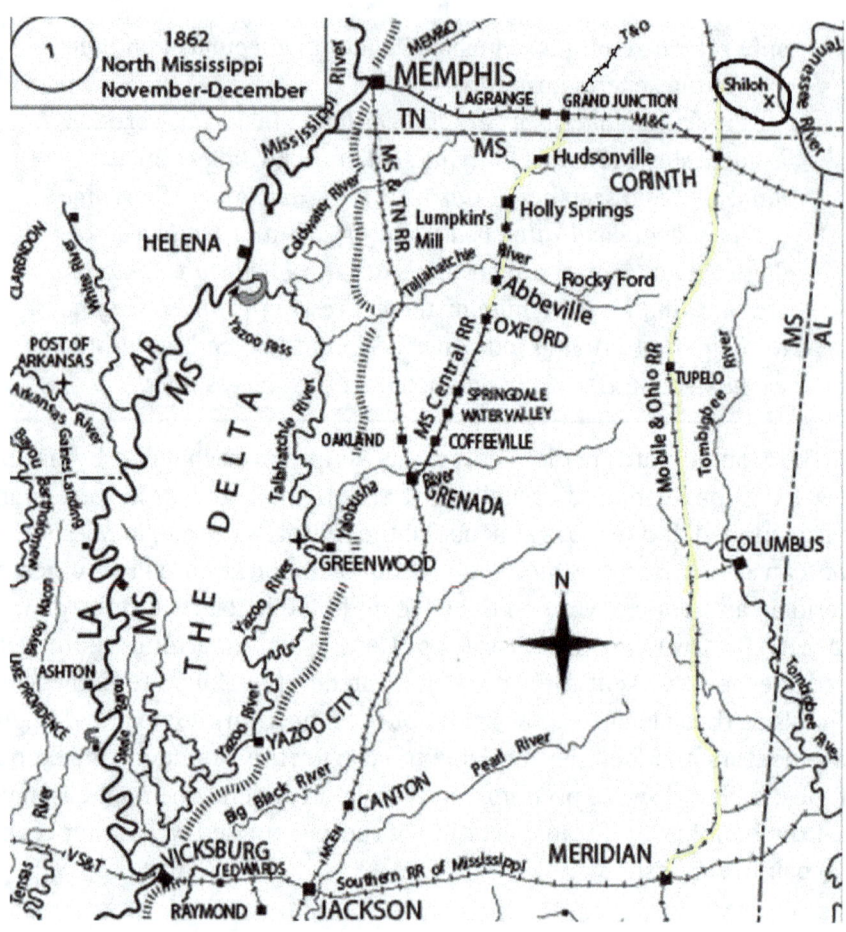

7-5: Northern Mississippi

CHAPTER 8
The Harris Car

In June 1862, Dr. Elisha Harris, of the U.S. Sanitary Commission, personally rode on one of the hospital trains using these improvised freight cars and witnessed the suffering caused by the jostling motion of the car. During the trip, Harris sketched out a system for hanging the stretchers with India rubber rings to serve as shock absorbers. He submitted his design for a hospital car to Quarter Master General Montgomery Meigs. He approved the plan and instructed the various railroads between Washington and New York City to begin altering existing passenger cars. He also ordered the USMRR to do the same thing in Alexandria, Virginia. Through the personal efforts of the Philadelphia, Wilmington and Baltimore Company's President Felton, the first such car was completed early in October 1862. The 51 foot long passenger car was fitted with upright posts to accommodate three tiers of berths. The genius of Dr. Harris's design was the fact that the patient never had to be removed from his stretcher. The soldier was taken from the field ambulances into the car and the poles of the stretcher inserted into huge rubber bands attached to the uprights.

The Harris car made it possible for the surgeon and other medical attendants to go from car to car while the train was in motion, something not possible in converted freight cars. However, the violent pitching and rolling of the moving train made treatment of the patients difficult. The rubber rings had the tendency to oscillate the bed while the train was moving, much to the annoyance of the patient. The more seriously wounded soldiers were place in the middle tiers so the surgeons could attend to them in case of an emergency. On the other hand, the design did allow for the same stretcher that carried a wounded soldier off of the battlefield to be used to transport him on the railcar and to serve as his bed in the general hospital, simplifying the loading and unloading of patients. It also made the process more comfortable for the patient by saving him from being lifted from one bed to another.

The "Harris car" could carry up to 36 recumbent patients and had seats at each end for the nurses or attendants. The cars were equipped with a stove, water tank, supply locker and toilet.

The following is only a small portion of a massive 9 by 32 foot mural painting by Anatoliy Shapiro. The painting is entitled *The Train Car*, and appears at the National Museum of Civil War Medicine in Frederick, Maryland. The 1999- 2000 Project was done with the assistance of two additional artists: Alexander Tkachenko and Barney Judge. The project included eight murals and dioramas which depicted camp life and medical treatment of the soldiers from both sides (Union and Confederate) during the Civil War.

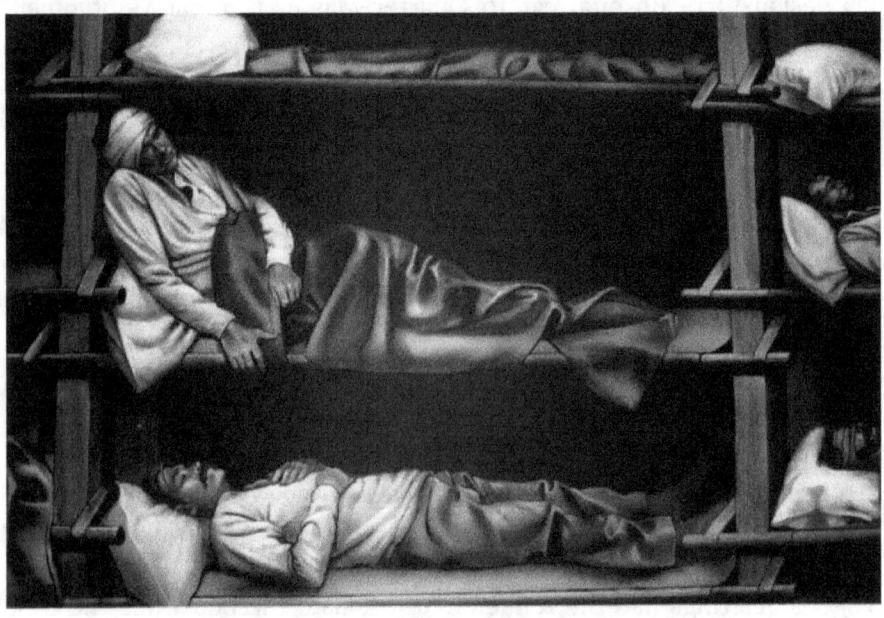

8-1: *The Train Car* by Anatoliy Shapiro. National Museum of Civil War Medicine, Frederick, Maryland.

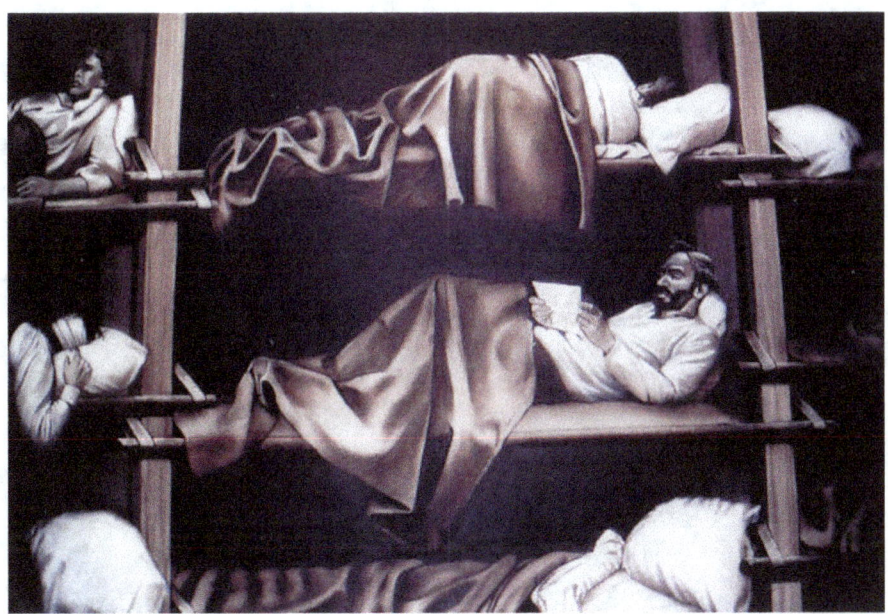

8-2: *The Train Car* by Anatoliy Shapiro. National Museum of Civil War Medicine, Frederick, Maryland.

As previously mentioned, in October 1862, Philadelphia, Wilmington and Baltimore Railroad was the first company to outfit and donate a hospital car configured to Harris's specifications. Fourteen cars were built with four placed in service, on regularly scheduled passenger trains, operating on the Louisville and Nashville Railroad line. This line was connected to hospitals in Louisville, Kentucky and Nashville, Tennessee serving General Grant's Army of the Tennessee.

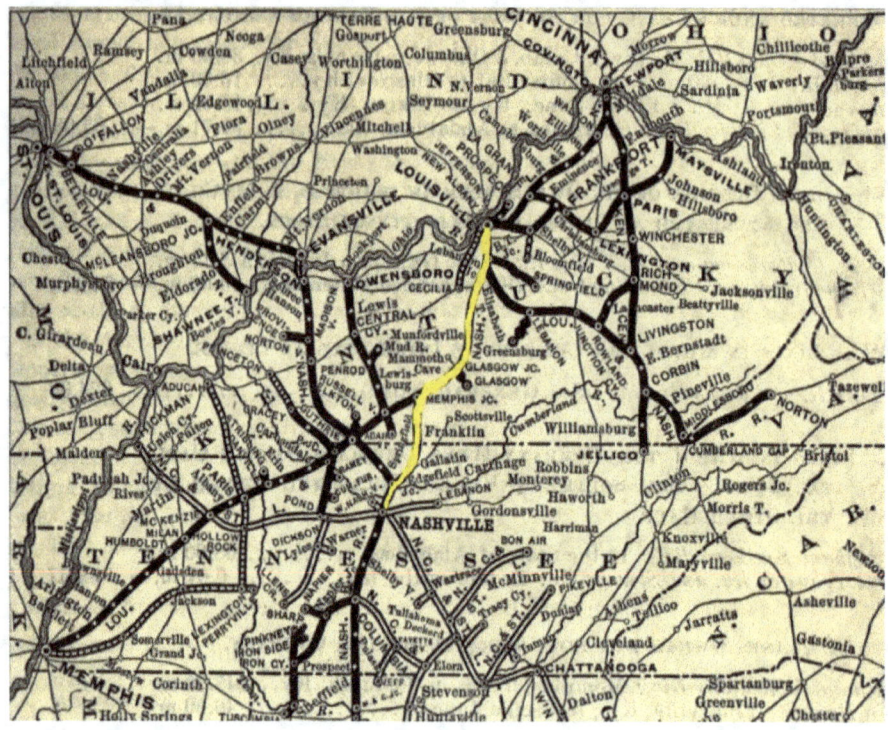

8-3: Louisville & Nashville Railroad Line

In the aftermath of the Battle of Perryville, fought on October 8, 1862, the U.S. Sanitary Commission utilized a Harris designed car in order to transport some of the more seriously wounded to Louisville, Kentucky, via the Louisville and Nashville Railroad line, where they were possibly treated at one or more of these hospitals: Brown (U.S. Army) or Clay, Crittenden or Foundry all which were serviced by volunteer groups. **For the North, It was their first regularly operated hospital car of the Civil War.**

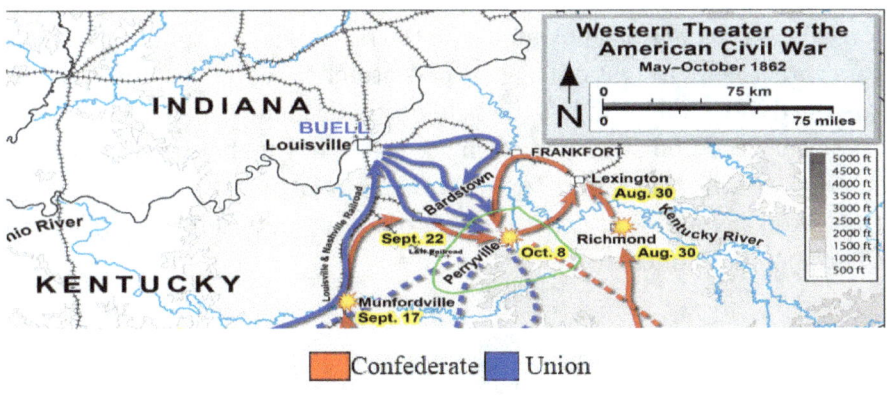

8-4: American Civil War Western Theater, May–October 1862

In the Harris designed car, thirty litters were suspended from rubber "tugs" which took up the jolts of railroad travel. A dispensary area provided medicines, towels, socks, and blankets while the kitchen area provided food, beverages and utensils. These cars were supplied, staffed and controlled by the U.S. Sanitary Commission which regularly operated on the Nashville-to-Louisville run throughout most of 1863.

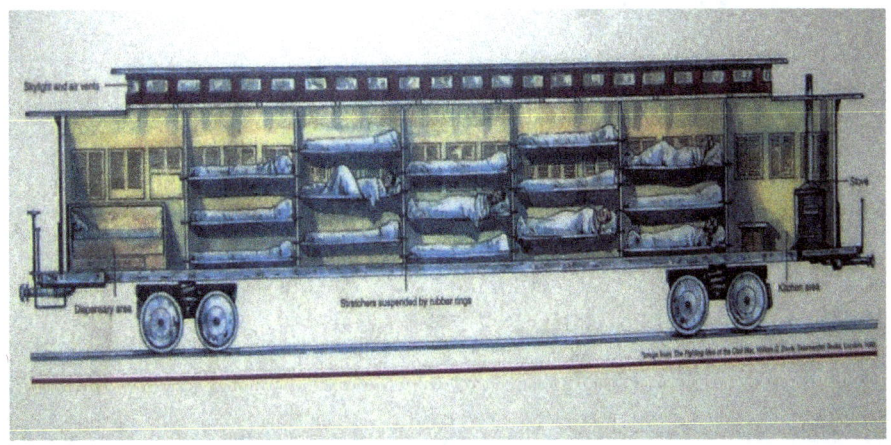

8-5: Harris US Hospital Railroad Car

These railcars reduced the travel time from Louisville to Nashville to 24 hours and were credited with preventing many cases of gangrene as was common on slower hospital ships. A journalist for *Harper's Weekly*, February 27, 1864, described the ride of the Harris hospital car as, "comfortable as the beds of a hospital." The Harris car was one of ten or twelve cars with several freight or baggage cars attached to the hospital car. This so-called "hospital train" left the field hospitals daily.

Besides the Louisville and Nashville Railroad run, between Louisville, Kentucky and Nashville, Tennessee, the Harris car was used on the Nashville and Chattanooga Railroad run between Nashville and Chattanooga, Tennessee.

CHAPTER 9

The United States Military Railroad

During the first six months of the war, with the Battles of Bull Run and Wilson's Creek still a harsh memory, the U.S. Army still continued to deal with railroads in an ad hoc manner. Since there was no official relationship between railroads and the Army, military officers, not understanding railroad operations, treated train crews as if they were teamsters. As a result, rail movements were not coordinated. Field units frequently used boxcars as warehouses. The most important event affecting the Union railroads occurred on January 31, 1862, not on a battlefield but in Congress. Congress passed a bill authorizing President Lincoln as Commander in Chief, "to take possession of any and all railroads and telegraph lines in the United States." Prior to this bill, administration of Union railroads had been in chaos. This was compounded by Simon Cameron who for the first year of the war was an inept and corrupt head of the War Department. Although the act was rarely used, railroad companies knew that if they did not cooperate they could be taken over by the government. About the same time, Edwin McMasters Stanton was appointed secretary of war. Stanton had been president of the Illinois Central Railroad. He established the United States Military Railroads (USMRR) to control Union railroads where necessary and operate railroads in the occupied South. In practice, however, the USMRR restricted its authority to Southern rail lines captured in the course of the war Colonel Daniel Craig McCallum was appointed director and superintendent.

When Edwin Stanton appointed Daniel McCallum superintendent of the United States Military Railroad he also appointed Herman Haupt as the North's Chief Railroad Engineer. From 1840 to 1847, Haupt was a professor of mathematics and engineering at Pennsylvania College. He drew the attention of J. Edgar Thomson who became chief engineer of the Pennsylvania Railroad. Haupt returned to the railroad business in 1847, accepting a position as construction engineer on the Pennsylvania Railroad, and then becoming its general superintendent from 1849 to 1851. Haupt and Thomson designed the Horseshoe Curve (now a National Historic Landmark) which enabled the Pennsylvania Railroad to cross the

Allegheny Mountains and reach Pittsburgh, Pennsylvania. From 1851 until 1853, Haupt was the chief engineer of the Southern Railroad of Mississippi, then became the Pennsylvania Railroad's chief engineer until 1856; in the latter position he completed the Mountain Division with the Allegheny Tunnel, opening the line through to Pittsburgh. He was the chief engineer on the five-mile (8 km) Hoosac Tunnel project through the Berkshires in Western Massachusetts from 1856 to 1861. No man had a greater effect on military railroads in the Civil War than Herman Haupt. He recruited an assortment of frontier woodsmen, skilled craftsman and freed slaves to create a railroad construction corps that achieved amazing engineering and railroad building feats. One of his first notable achievements was the reconstruction of the bridge over Potomac Creek. The original bridge took three years to build. Haupt and his men rebuilt the 300 foot long and 100 foot tall trestle in less than a week. Abraham Lincoln, amazed upon seeing the bridge, commented, "that man Haupt has built a bridge using bean-poles and cornstalks." In his Alexandria, Virginia headquarters Haupt also developed prefabricated components to rapidly repair destroyed bridges as well as field methods to efficiently repair or destroy track. Although Haupt served the Union Army for only fifteen months, he nevertheless left an indelible mark on the Northern rail system. At the time of the Civil War he was the best known railroad construction engineer in American.

The United States Military Railroad | 61

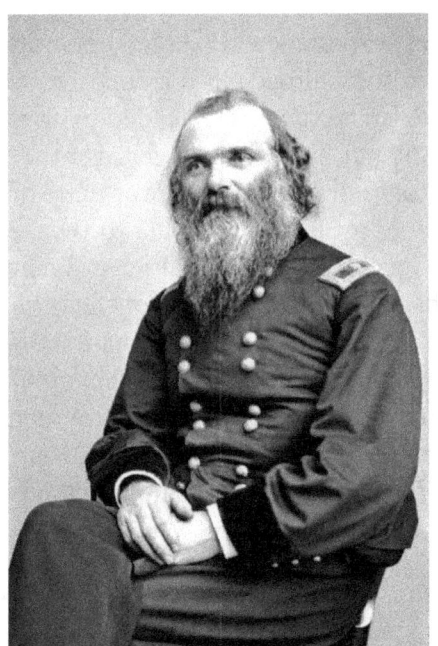

9-1: Daniel Craig McCallum

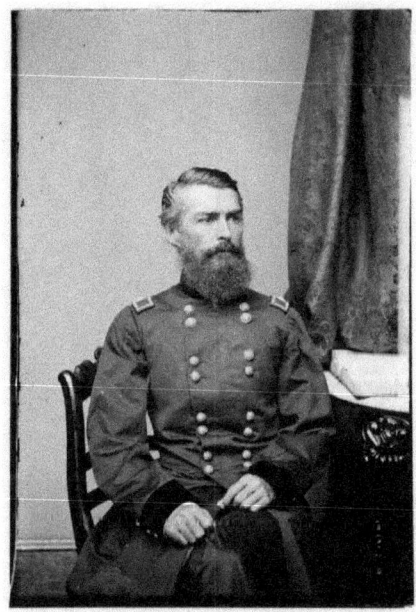

9-2: Herman Haupt

Both men had vast experience in railroad operations and were able to rebuild and organize the railroads into a cohesive system that provided the U.S. Army the logistical support it needed to ultimately win the war.

Jefferson Davis did not have such power over the conduct of the railroad in the South. To properly conduct a war there must be a centralized authority. That concept was an anathema to the Confederate cause of state's rights and decentralized federal government. Railroad companies in the South had such little respect for the government they would sometimes charge military rates higher than those charged civilians. During the war three men, William Ashe, William Wadley and Frederick Sims were placed in charge of Confederate railroads. Each would find his task impossible due to his lack of authority. Not until February 1865, would the Confederate Congress give Jefferson Davis control of the then it was too late.

CHAPTER 10
The Peninsula Campaign

The Peninsula Campaign was a major Union operation launched in southeastern Virginia from March 17, 1862 through the start of the Battle of Seven Pines on May 31, 1862. It was the first large-scale offensive in the Eastern Theater of the Civil War. The operation, under the leadership of Major General George B. McClellan, was an amphibious turning movement against the forces of the Confederate States Army in Northern Virginia. Its ultimate objective was to capture the Confederate capital of Richmond. McClellan was initially successful against the equally cautious General Joseph E. Johnston, but the active entry of the more aggressive General Robert E. Lee turned the tide in this campaign ending in a humiliating Union retreat and withdrawal from the field of battle.

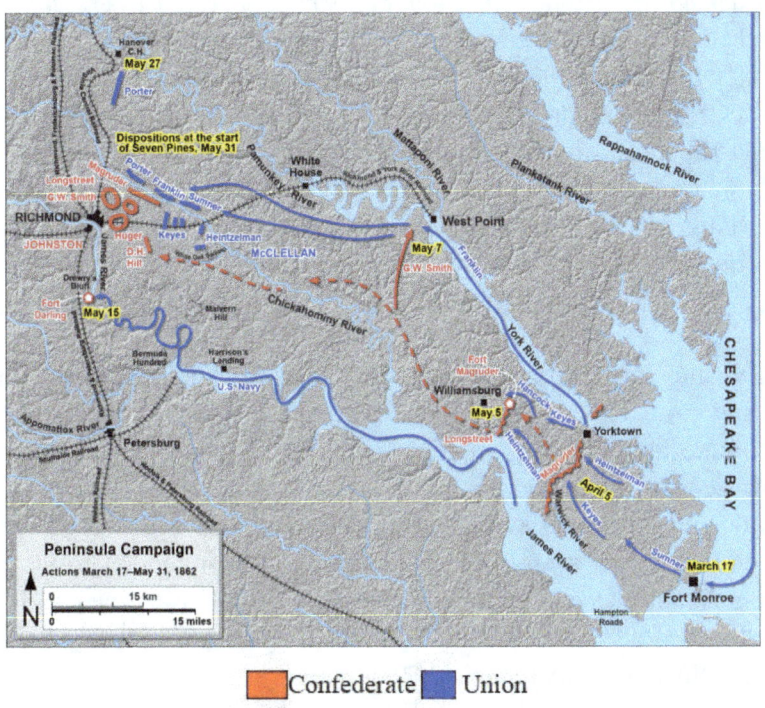

10-1: Peninsula Campaign, March 17 - May 31, 1862

The U.S. Sanitary Commission, at the request of the army, created the Hospital Transport Service. It acquired 16 medium and large boats and converted them to hospital ships. Its first major operations came in the Peninsular Campaign of spring 1862, when it serviced casualties from General McClellan's Army of 100,000 men after a series of battles. The Sanitary Commission quickly organized large fleets of ships and created a network system of routes to move wounded. By mid-May, the Commission's Hospital Transport Service had seven ships working out of White House Landing, Virginia on the York River and Harrison's Landing on the James River. The Service ended with the end of the Peninsula Campaign in July 1862.

The reason for the creation of the Hospital Transport Service is explained in the book Women's Work in the Civil War:

> "...in April, 1862, the 'Hospital Transport Service' was organized, principally by the efforts of Mr. Frederick Law Olmstead, the General Secretary of the Sanitary Commission. The sudden transfer of the scene of active war from the high grounds bordering the Potomac to a low and swampy region intersected by a network of creeks and rivers, made necessary appliances for the care of the sick and wounded, which the Government was not at that time prepared to furnish. Hence arose the arrangement by which certain large steamers, chartered, but then unemployed by the Government, were transferred to the Sanitary Commission to be fitted up as Hospital Transports for the reception and conveyance of the sick and wounded.
> --Women's Work in the Civil War

Each ship carried upwards of several hundred soldiers, many of them suffering from various diseases. Tending to the sick and wounded on board were female nurses, many of whom had followed their husbands who were working as doctors.

The Sanitary Commission quickly organized large fleets of ships and created a network system of routes to move wounded. Various rivers and the Atlantic Ocean connecting became the highway over which the wounded steadily traveled further North. The Service ended with the end of the Peninsula Campaign in July 1862.

A number of hospital ships, including the *Empress, Imperial, Daniel Webster 2, Ocean Queen,* and the *Wilson Small* embarked at various, including White House Landing on the Pamunkey River and Harrison's Landing on the James River. They transported the wounded to hospitals in Fortress Monroe, including the Chesapeake Hospital.

Here are images of the *Daniel Webster 2* and *Ocean Queen* which plied the inland waters of Virginia in order to transport the sick and wounded from battles during the 1862 Peninsula Campaign.

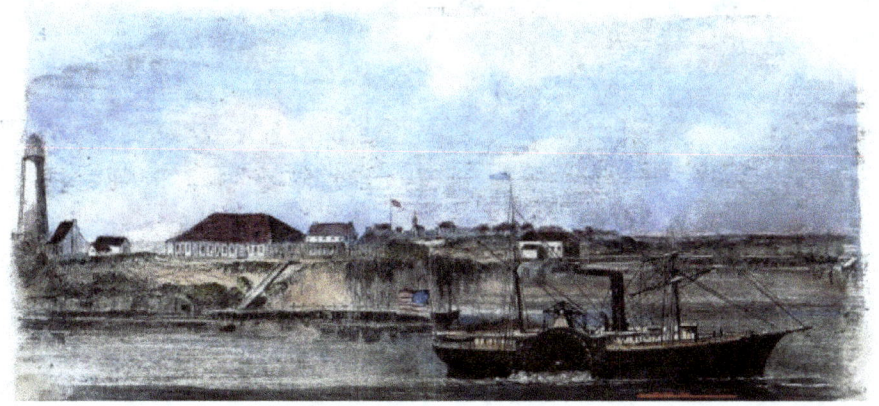

10-2: Hospital Transport Ship *Daniel Webster 2*

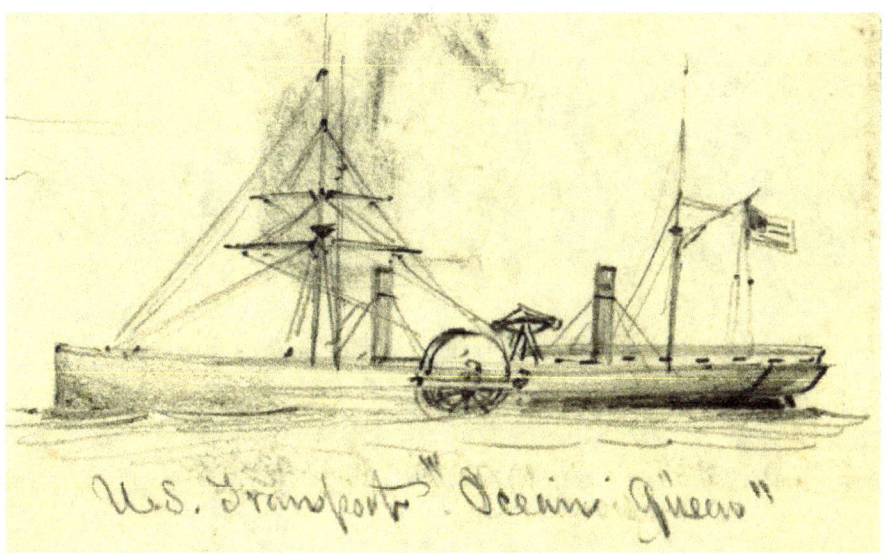

10-3: Hospital Transport Ship *Ocean Queen*

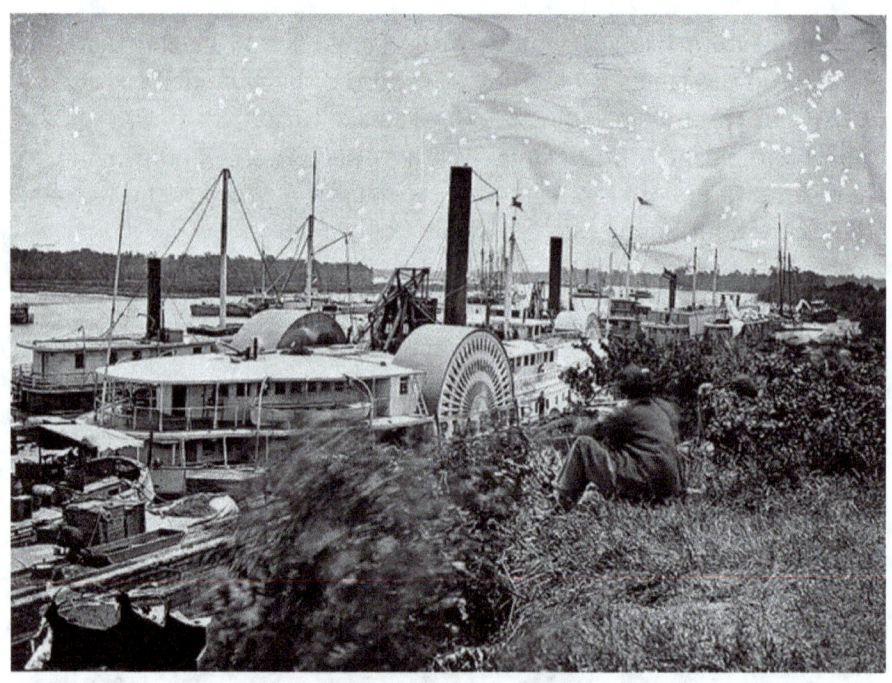

10-4: White House Landing on the Pamunkey River.

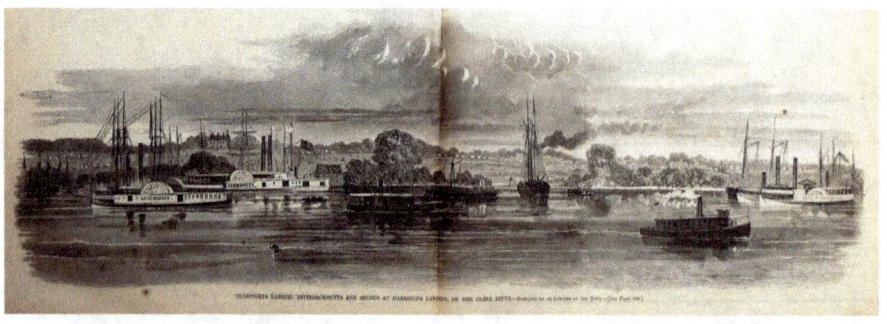

10-5: Port facilities at Harrison's Landing, on the James River.

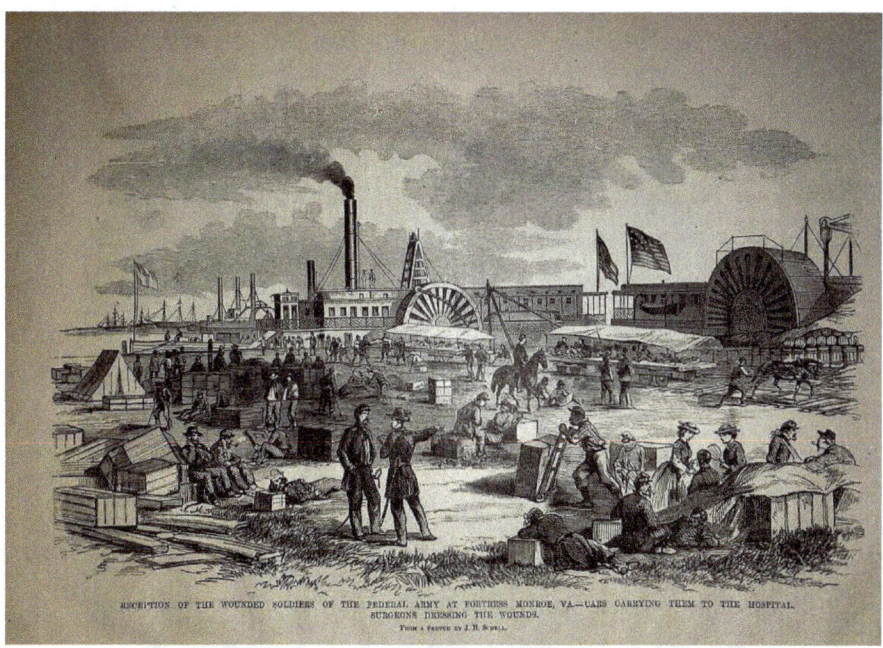

10-6: Wounded soldiers removed from hospital ships. Surgeons are dressing their wounds before these wounded are conveyed to one of the hospitals at Fortress Monroe by covered, horse-drawn, flat railcars.

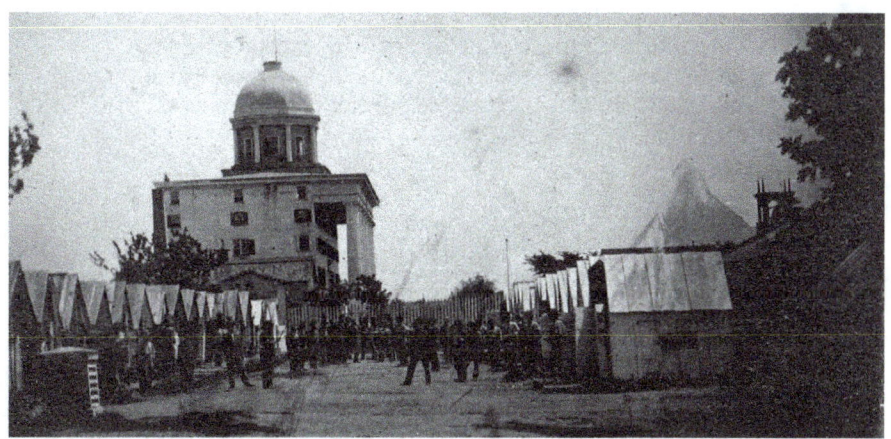

10-7: Chesapeake Hospital located at Fortress Monroe.

Other vessels embarked from Fortress Monroe, disembarking at the DeCamp General Hospital on Davids' Island, New York. Their voyage took seven days to complete.

These included the Hospital Transport S.R. *Spaulding* and the *Daniel Webster 1*.

2658, HOSPITAL TRANSPORT S.R. SPAULDING.

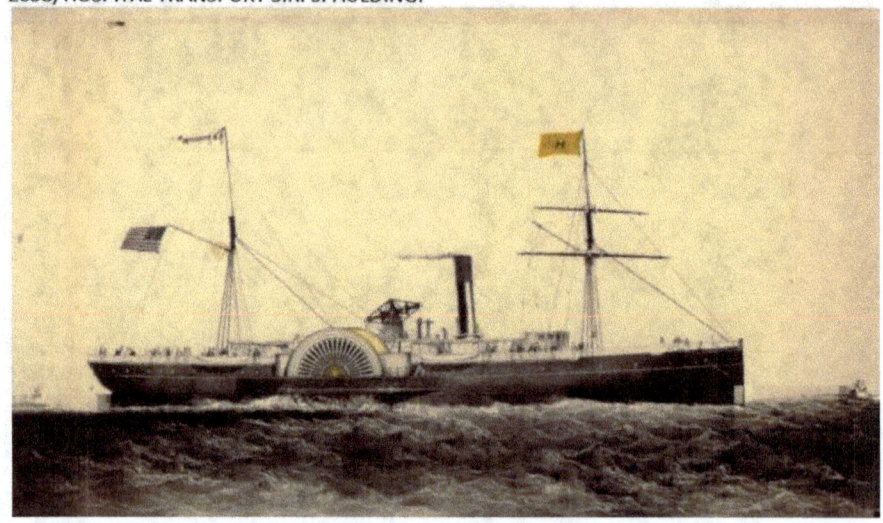

10-8: Hospital Transport Ship *Spaulding*, described in the book Hospital Transports: "...a large, seaworthy vessel... She was fitted for carrying cavalry, with stalls for horses, and at this time filled with stable odor, and needed coal and water as well as complete interior reconstruction."

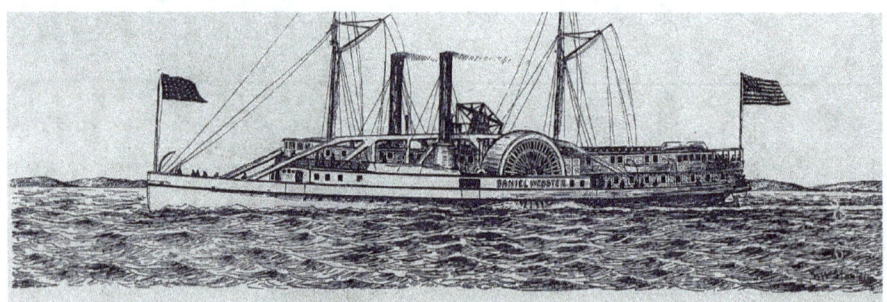

10-9: Hospital Transport Ship *Daniel Webster 1*

Finally, other hospital ships embarked at White House Landing on the Pamunkey River and disembarked principally in Philadelphia, a voyage of six days, Washington, D.C. and Baltimore, a voyage of four days. These vessels, with a capacity of 400-450 patients, included the *Elm City*, *Vanderbilt*, *Louisiana*, and *State of Maine*. On June 27, 1862, after an untold number of voyages transporting the wounded, the *Elm City* and the other aforementioned hospital ships were no longer able to use White House Landing. The place was, during most of the Peninsular Campaign, the main base of supplies for the Army of the Potomac. Previously a backwater, it had been transformed into a bustling river port. But on June 27, that all changed. On that day, with the Union defeat at the Battle of Gaines' Mill, sometimes known as the Battle of Chickahominy River. General McClellan made the decision to abandon White House Landing and change his base to Harrison Landing on the James River. Everything at White House Landing was thrown into panic and chaos.

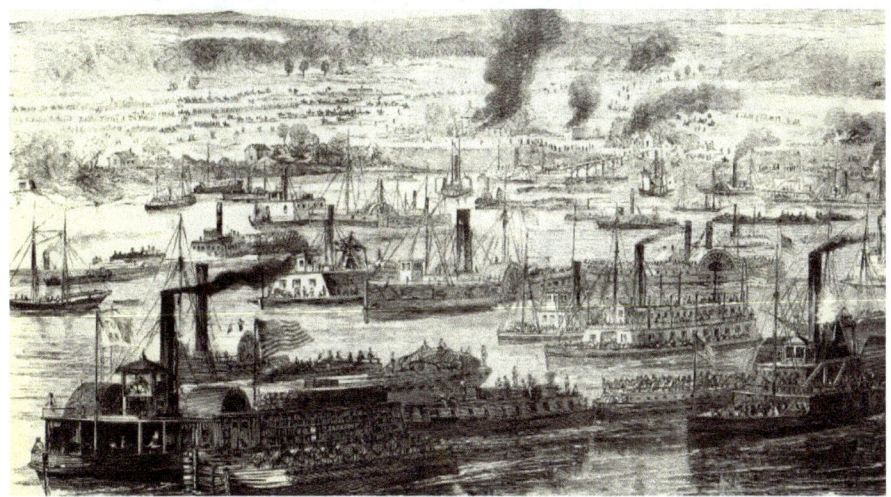

10-10: White House Landing

Katherine Wormeley wrote aboard the *Elm City*:

> "...General Porter, being flanked in immense force, has wheeled round and back...The whole army is now across the [Chickahominy] river; the enemy are in part on this side of it... The enemy evidently hope to ruin us by seizing this station... Everything has been sent away; the few things that remain are

lying on the wharves... The Elm City is waiting for the 93rd New York Regiment, which is stationed here on guard duty... Even as I write comes the order to start, the enemy having got the railroad. And so rapidly have we gone, that between writing the words 'Elm City' and 'railroad' we are off! Such a jolly panic! Men rushing and tearing down to the wharves... The enemy are in force three miles from us; they have seized the railroad, and cut the telegraph."

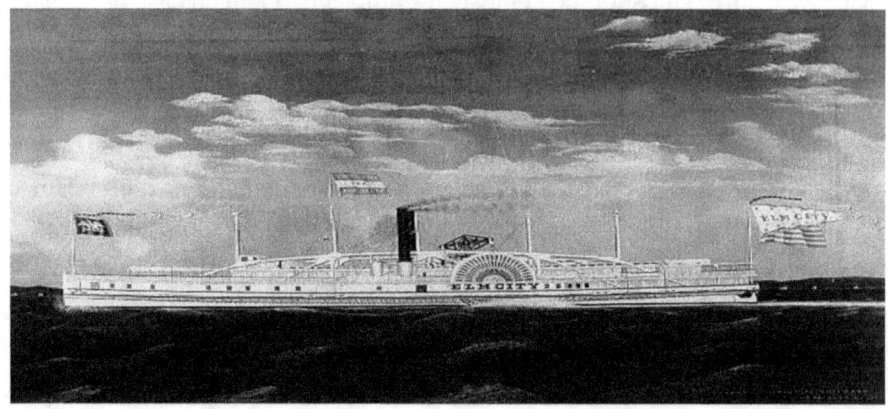

10-11: Hospital Transport Ship *Elm City*

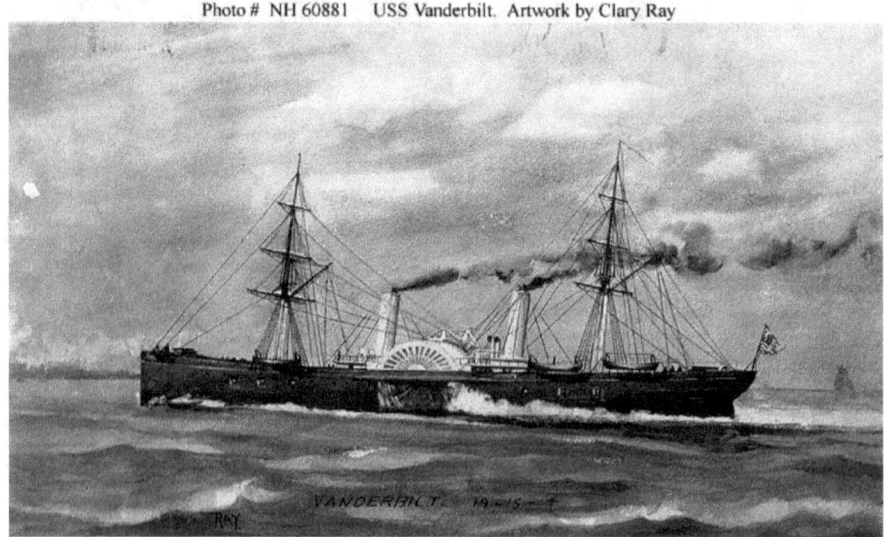

10-12: Hospital Transport Ship *Vanderbilt*

lying on the wharves... The Elm City is waiting for the 93rd New York Regiment, which is stationed here on guard duty... Even as I write comes the order to start, the enemy having got the railroad. And so rapidly have we gone, that between writing the words 'Elm City' and 'railroad' we are off! Such a jolly panic! Men rushing and tearing down to the wharves... The enemy are in force three miles from us; they have seized the railroad, and cut the telegraph."

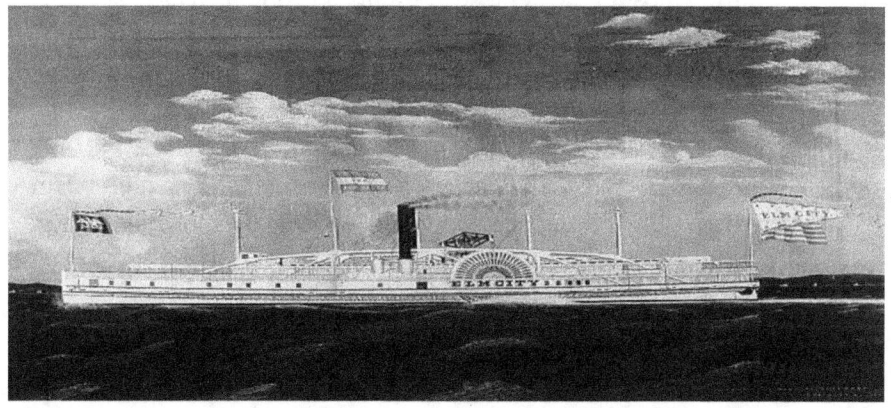

10-11: Hospital Transport Ship *Elm City*

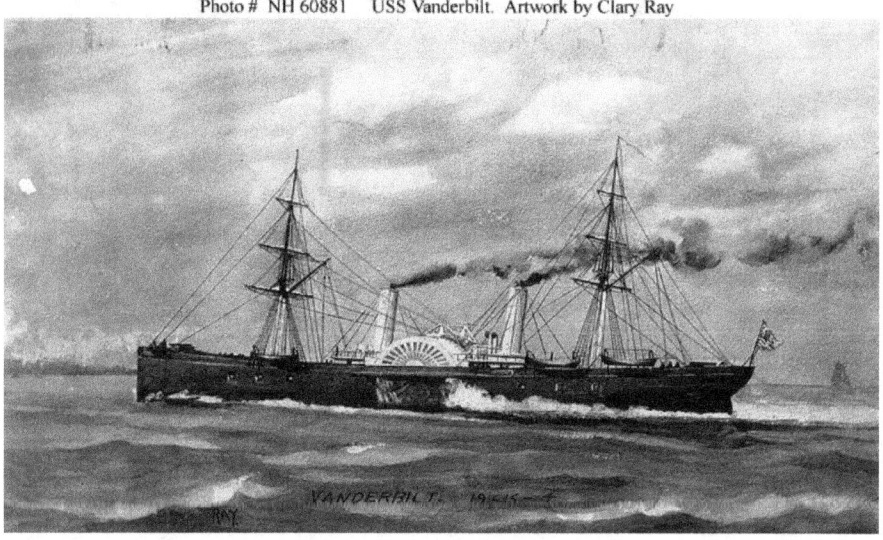

10-12: Hospital Transport Ship *Vanderbilt*

Finally, other hospital ships embarked at White House Landing on the Pamunkey River and disembarked principally in Philadelphia, a voyage of six days, Washington, D.C. and Baltimore, a voyage of four days. These vessels, with a capacity of 400-450 patients, included the *Elm City*, *Vanderbilt*, *Louisiana*, and *State of Maine*. On June 27, 1862, after an untold number of voyages transporting the wounded, the *Elm City* and the other aforementioned hospital ships were no longer able to use White House Landing. The place was, during most of the Peninsular Campaign, the main base of supplies for the Army of the Potomac. Previously a backwater, it had been transformed into a bustling river port. But on June 27, that all changed. On that day, with the Union defeat at the Battle of Gaines' Mill, sometimes known as the Battle of Chickahominy River. General McClellan made the decision to abandon White House Landing and change his base to Harrison Landing on the James River. Everything at White House Landing was thrown into panic and chaos.

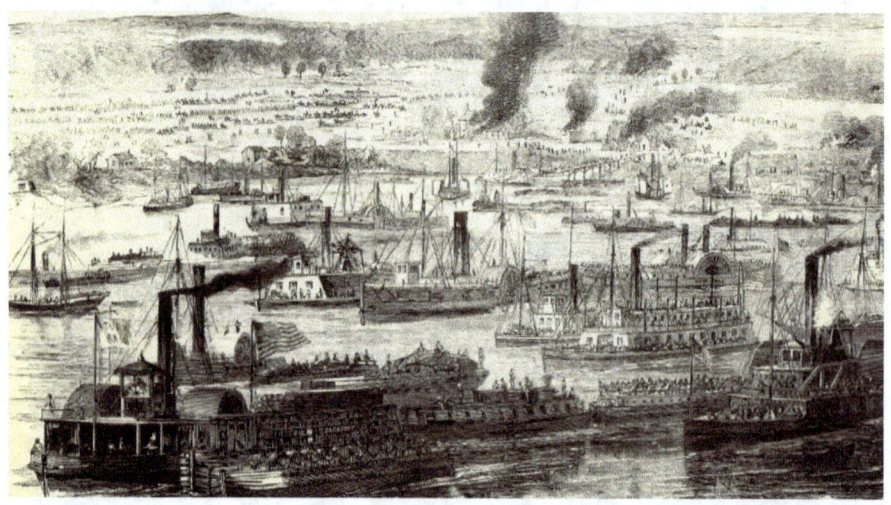

10-10: White House Landing

Katherine Wormeley wrote aboard the *Elm City*:

> "...*General Porter, being flanked in immense force, has wheeled round and back...The whole army is now across the [Chickahominy] river; the enemy are in part on this side of it... The enemy evidently hope to ruin us by seizing this station... Everything has been sent away; the few things that remain are*

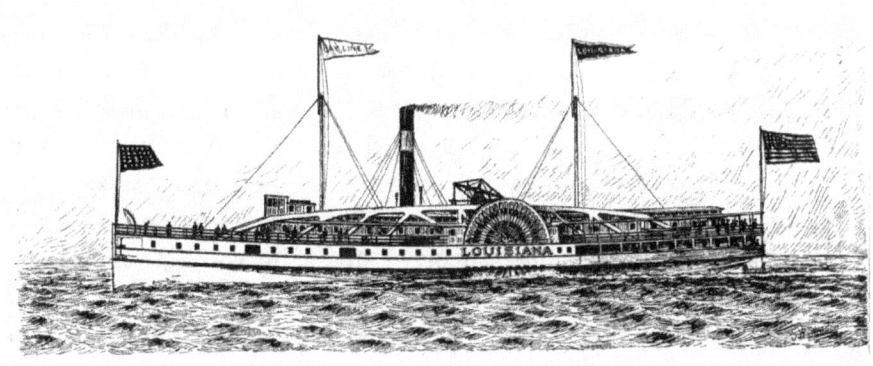

CHESAPEAKE BAY STEAMBOAT LOUISIANA, 1854.

10-13: Hospital Transport Ship *Louisiana*

The *Louisiana* was typical of these ocean going hospital ships transporting the sick and wounded in the Eastern Theater. The boat was divided into four wards, two on the lower deck and two on the upper or boiler deck, each of which had a medical officer, a ward master, six permanently detailed male nurses, and one female nurse. The nurses were relieved from duty every six hours, day and night. Upon the lower deck was the kitchen, commissary, storeroom, bakery, and ice-house; upon the upper deck the captain's office was converted into the office of the Surgeon in charge, and the bar-room into a dispensary, the barber-shop and wash-room into a kitchen for low and half-diet patients under the supervision of a female nurse. The bulkheads between the state-rooms were removed, improving the ventilation and rendering access to the patients easier. Beds were also placed on the guards of the boat, tarpaulins being stretched to protect the patients from the inclement weather. The texas upon the hurricane deck was used as quarters for the hospital attendants and the boat's crew. An oven was on board capable of baking bread for a thousand men daily. In admitting as well as in removing the patients a systematic arrangement was adopted. A medical officer was stationed at the gangway to receive them, one on the boiler, and another on the lower deck. Each ward master remained in his ward, and a sufficient number of nurses was detailed to carry the patients on or off the boat. By this arrangement all confusion was avoided; no one was admitted as a patient except upon a written order from the Medical Director.

The boat at this time had accommodations for four hundred patients. In April 1863, the boat was purchased by the Government and remodeled as a permanent hospital boat, with beds for four hundred and fifty patients, and was named the *R. C. Wood*, in honor of the Assistant Surgeon General of the United States Army, to whose wisdom, humanity, and constant foresight many of the improvements in the hospital arrangements were due. Surgeon T. F. Azpell, U. S. V., was placed in charge. Her state-rooms were removed, the whole upper deck was made into one large ward, with abundant light and excellent means of ventilation, with ample provisions of bath-rooms, hot and cold water, cooking apartments, nurses' rooms, dispensary, laundry, and many other conveniences. Her length was two hundred and fifty feet, beam forty feet, hold seven feet. From April 1863, to April 11, 1865, this boat made thirty-three trips, travelled thirty-four thousand eight hundred and five miles, and carried eleven thousand and twenty-four (11,024) sick and wounded exclusively in the Western Theater.

2660,HOSPITAL STEAMER STATE OF MAINE.

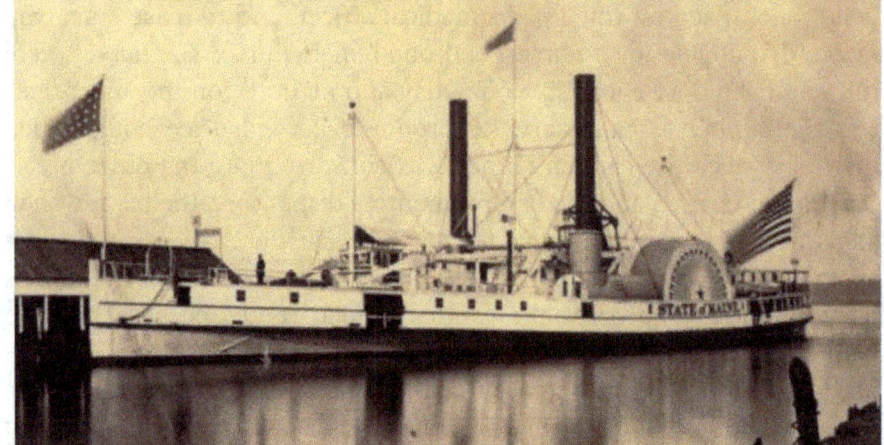

10-14: Hospital Transport Ship *State of Maine*

Clara Jones, a full-time teacher, had some remarkable wartime experiences which included assisting the wounded aboard a hospital ship, and at hospitals in Alexandria, Virginia, and at Gettysburg, Pennsylvania.

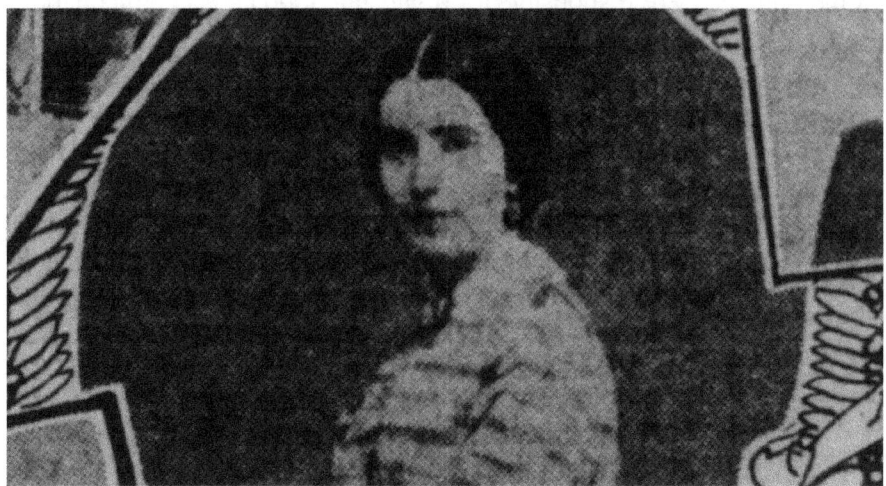

10-15: Clara Jones

When school closed on July 9, 1862 and by August, Jones had started full-time hospital work aboard a boat, the *State of Maine*. Over the month of August, the *State of Maine* transported more than 3,000 sick soldiers from the Virginia Peninsula.

Her relief efforts on the ship typically involved offering the soldiers comforting food and drink:

> "The supply of wine and jelly contributed by my dear girls was found very acceptable as were the pickles which I, myself, distributed among them... I saw men sit down and cry like children to find themselves once more under the protection of our flag, and receiving the comfort that they had so longed for."

Female nurses were most welcomed on the Sanitary Commission's Hospital Transport Service's hospital ships. These ships, launched in the spring of 1862 in coordination with McClellan's campaign against the Confederacy in Virginia, brought injured soldiers home off of the battlefield. While the Army had had difficulties accepting female nurses at the hospitals on land, Sanitary Commissioner Frederick Law Olmstead, who organized the ships, wanted to bring women aboard as nurses because they could provide a "home away from home" for the sick and injured soldiers. His vision was in line with the notion of the female "domestic sphere." These women nurses were responsible for organizing food and accommodations on board, tending to soldiers' needs, and assisting the medical staff.

Ellen (nicknamed ellie) Ruggles Strong served as a chief nurse aboard U.S. Sanitary Commission Hospital Transport Service ships in support of the Peninsula Campaign. These ships transported the wounded from this campaign to general hospitals in Washington, D.C., Philadelphia and New York City. As observed in the *Women's Work in the Civil War: A Record of Heroism, Patriotism and Patience*, written by L.P. Brockett and Mrs. Mary C. Vaughan:

> *"Among those who were in charge of the Hospital Transports for one or more of their trips to the cities we have named, and by the tenderness and gentleness comforted and cheered the poor sufferers, and often by their skillful nursing rescued them from the jaws of death, were Mrs. George T. Strong, the wife of the Treasurer of the Commission, who made four or five trips..."*

In *The Diary of George Templeton Strong, Vol. 3: The Civil War, 1860-1865*, dated June 12, 1862, George Templeton Strong writes of Ellie, his wife, and her interest in nursing Union sick and wounded:

> *"Her capacity of unselfishness and intense desire to employ it constitute a 'call' to this humane and patriotic womanly work . . . which I cannot but hear, though unwillingly."*

From the script of Ken Burns epic documentary film *The Civil War*:

> *"[George Templeton Strong's wife, Ellie, went south to serve on a hospital ship, too]... Ellie's tact, sense, good nature, and energy conquered the USA surgeon in charge at once, and coerced all his official dignity into hearty, grateful cooperation in the care of his cargo of 500 'cases,' mostly bad ones. I have never given her credit for tithe of the enterprise, pluck, discretion and force of character she has shown. God bless her..."*

These nurses "set aside traditional feminine values and clothing, and even went as far as to copy a flannel shirt stolen from a Dr. Agnew." They wore these "Agnews" with their skirts. Also assigned to the Hospital Transport Service, as a nurse, was Katherine Wormeley. She is quoted as saying:

> "When there wasn't enough equipment on the ship to make the hundreds of meals necessary, the women crept off the ship and stole a stove from a general's quarters... Kleptomania is the prevailing disease among us... We think nothing of watching the proprietor of some nicety out of the way, and then pocketing the article."

The women believed their work to be vitally important. Wormeley said later:

> "...we worked together under the deepest feelings, and to the extent of our powers, shoulder to shoulder, helping each other to the best of our ability, and no one failing or hindering another." Olmstead was proud of the women as well: "God knows what we should have done without them, they have worked like heroes night and day, and though the duty is frequently most disagreeable ... I have never seen one of them flinch for a moment."

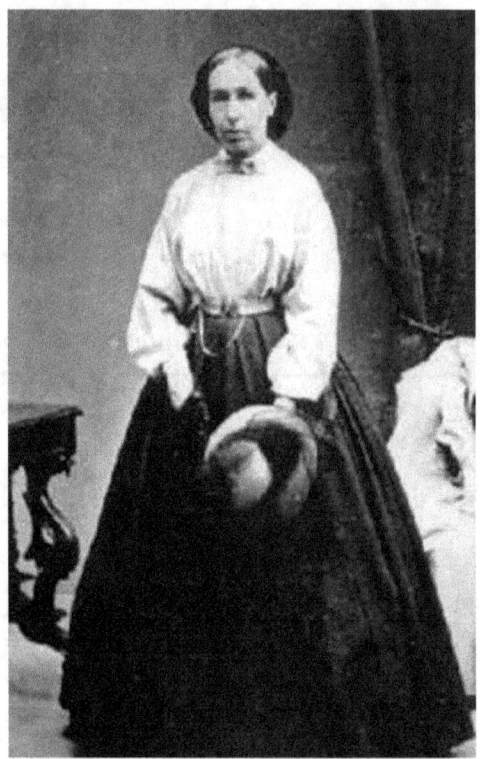

10-16: Katherine Prescott Wormeley in her "Agnew" Shirt

In her book, *The Other Side of War with the Army of the Potomac*, she describes the origins, duties, and early work of the newly-formed United States Sanitary Commission. "It was the outgrowth of a demand made by the women of the country" because both men and women wanted to contribute to the war effort. "As the men mustered for the battlefield, so the women mustered in churches, schoolhouses, and parlors...."

By May 10, she scripted her writing from the *Daniel Webster* 2, a floating hospital. The vessel could handle up to 300 wounded soldiers and embarked them on the Pamunkey River. As one of four women on the ship, her duties were "very much that of a housekeeper." She had just received, stowed, and fed 245 men, most ill with typhoid fever. As each man came aboard, "I gave him brandy and water," and later, tea, bread and butter. The "fever patients are very dreadful, and their moans are distressing. The men were all patient and grateful. Some said, 'You don't know what it is to me to see you... To think of a woman being here to help me!'"

In a subsequent letter she describes a normal day on the ship:

> "I took my first actual watch last night... We begin the day by getting them all washed, and freshened up, and breakfasted. Then the surgeons and dressers make their rounds, open the wounds, apply the remedies, and replace the bandages. This is an awful hour; I sat with my fingers in my ears this morning.
>
> "The horrors of that morning are too great to speak of. The men in the cars were brought on board the Daniel Webster 2 and laid about the vacant main-deck and guards and on the deck of a scow that lay alongside. I must not, I ought not to tell you of the horrors of that morning. One of the least was that I saw a "contraband" (Author's note: contraband, in this case, refers to an escaped slave during the Civil War who fled to or was taken behind Union lines) step on the amputated stump of a wretched man. I took him by the arm and walked him into the tent, where I ordered them to give him other work, and forbade that he should come upon the ships again. I felt white with anger, and dared not trust myself to speak to him. While those awful sights pass before me I have comparatively no feeling, except the anxiety to alleviate as much as possible. I do not suffer under the sights; but oh! the sounds, the screams of men. It is when I think of it afterwards that it is so dreadful..."

Sanitary Commission volunteer Georgeanna Woolsey recorded her observations aboard a hospital ship, involved in the Peninsula Campaign in *My Heart Toward Home: Letters of a Family During the Civil War*, by Georgeanna Woolsey Bacon and Eliza Woolsey Howland. In a letter to her mother in 1862 from the hospital ship *Ocean Queen* off the coast of Virginia. Georgy Woolsey wrote:

> "The immense saloon of the after-cabin was filled with mattresses so thickly placed that there was hardly stepping room between them, and as I swung my lantern along a row of pale faces, it showed me another strong dead man... We are all changed by this contact with terror, else how could I deliberately turn my lantern on his face and say to the Doctor behind me, 'Is that man dead?' And stand coolly while he listened and

examined and pronounced him dead. I could not have said quietly a year ago, 'That will make one more bed then, Doctor.'"

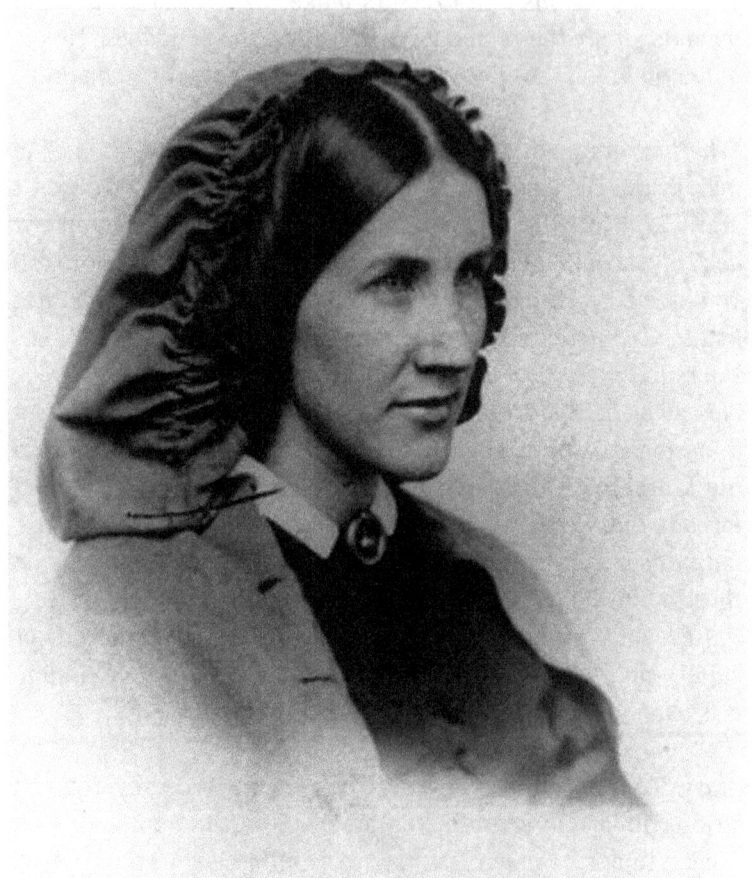

10-17: Georgeanna Woolsey

The *Ocean Queen* had a capacity of 400 patients and transported the wounded from Janes River to Fortress Monroe, a journey of 2 days.

CHAPTER 11
The Battle of Seven Pines

The Battle of Seven Pines, also known as the Battle of Fair Oaks by the Confederacy, took place on May 31 and June 1, 1862, in Henrico County, Virginia, and was part of the Peninsula Campaign.

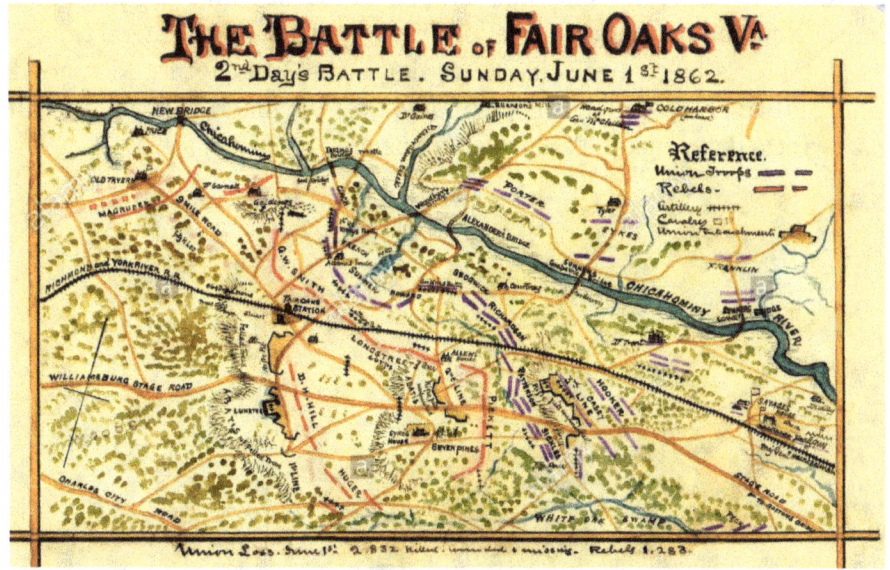

11-1: The Battle of Seven Pines (Battle of Fair Oaks),
color rendition of original sketch by Arthur Lumley

It was a two-day battle in which numerous Confederate attacks were repulsed. The battle was fought just six miles east of the Confederate capital at Richmond, Virginia. The Union Army of the Potomac was under the command of Major General George B. McClellan and the Confederate forces were led by General Joseph E. Johnston. The general was severely wounded in the first day of fighting. Northern casualties numbered more than 5,000 while Southern casualties numbered more than 6,000.

Arthur Lumley's sketch shows the Ambulance Corps carrying and loading wounded Union soldiers onto rail cars of the Richmond and York

River Railroad following the Battle of Seven Pines which is was called the Battle of Fair Oaks (May 31-June 1, 1862) by the Confederacy. Although this railroad originally operated within the Confederacy, the Union Army took possession of it early in the war. The cars would be covered with straw and blankets, and a gangplank made the transfer easier. The patients suffered an excruciating ride in the four-wheeled ambulance shown in the center of the sketch. Branches were cut and fixed to the flatcars to provide some shade for the wounded. The locomotive pictured here is the Exetor. The railroad was founded on January 31, 1853 and operated 39 miles (63 km) of railroad line between Richmond, Virginia and West Point, Virginia on the York River. The railroad was a key strategic goal of Union General George B. McClellan's failed Peninsula Campaign in 1862 to capture Richmond. The railroad prospered during the first year of the American Civil War but was wrecked during the Peninsula Campaign.

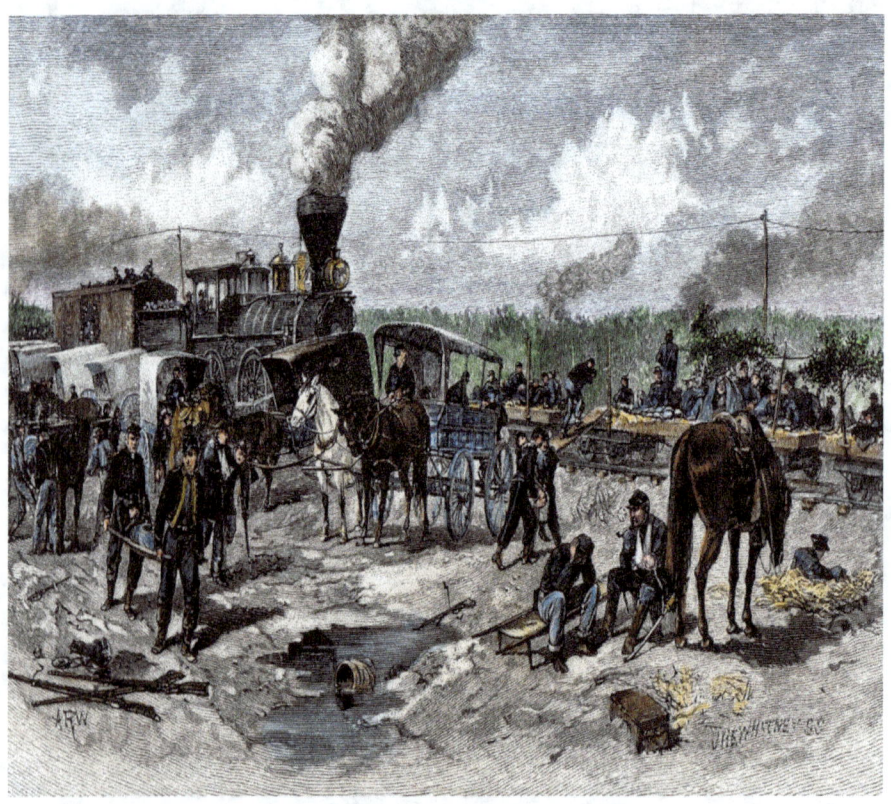

11-2: Richmond & York River Railroad

The railroad was founded on January 31, 1853 and operated 39 miles (63 km) of railroad line between Richmond, Virginia and West Point, Virginia on the York River. However, in order to expedite their evacuation, these wounded soldiers would disembark at the White House Landing where the railroad first crosses the Pamunkey River. At this location, an Army evacuation hospital, consisting of 105 hospital tents, had been established in order to "stabilize" the wounded before they were transported by steamers which were used as hospital ships.

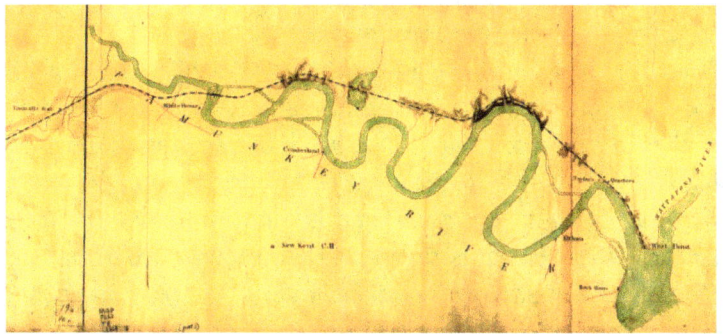

11-3: York River

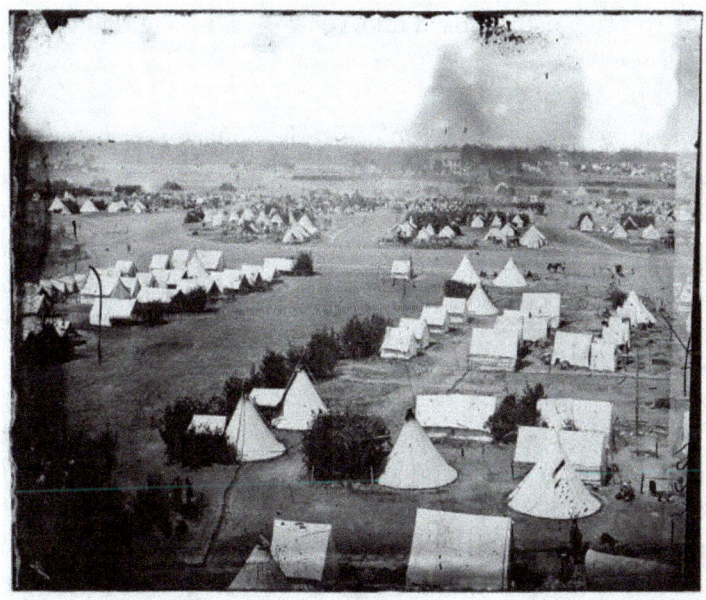

11-4: Hospital Tents

Mrs. John Harris, the wife of a prominent physician in Philadelphia, served first aboard the hospital ship *Vanderbilt* following the Battle of Fair Oaks. Here is an account of her recollections as related in the book *Women's Work in the Civil War: A Record of Heroism, Patriotism and Patience*, written by L.P. Brockett and Mrs. Mary C. Vaughan:

> "...From thence [Mrs. Harris] went on board the Vanderbilt, then just taken as a Government Transport for the wounded from the bloody field of Fair Oaks.
> "She thus describes the scene and her work:
> 'There were eight hundred on board. Passage-ways, state-rooms, floors from the dark and foetid hold to the hurrican deck, were all more than filled; some on mattresses, some on blankets, others on straw; some in the death-struggle, others nearing it, some already beyond human sympathy and help; some in their blood as they had been brought from the battle-field of the Sabbath previous, and all hungry and thirsty, not having had anything to eat or drink, except hard crackers, for twenty-four hours.'"

On the afternoon of the next day (or the next but one), Mrs. Harris describes the scenes on board another vessel, in like manner freighted with suffering.

> "The afternoon found us on board the Louisiana, where fearful sights met us. The whole day had been spent in operating. In one pile lay seventeen arms, hands, feet, and legs. A large proportion of the wounded had undergone mutilation in some important member. Many must die. Four lay with their faces covered, dying or dead. Many had not had their wounds dressed since the battle, and were in a sad state already. One brave fellow, from Maine, had lost both legs, and bore up with wonderful firmness. Upon my saying to him, 'You have suffered much for your country; we cannot thank you enough,' he replied, 'O, well, you hadn't ought to thank me. I went of my own accord, in a glorious cause. God bless McClellan.'
> "And here let me say, the young lady, Miss B., whom I brought with me, spent the whole of Friday night on board the Louisiana,

dressing and caring for the wounded. When I left the boat, at eleven o'clock at night, I was obliged to wash all my skirts, being drabbled in the mingled blood of Federal and Confederate soldiers, which covered many portions of the floor. I was obliged to kneel between them to wash their faces. This is war."

CHAPTER 12
The Battle of Savage's Station

The Battle of Savage's Station took place on June 29, 1862, in Henrico County, Virginia, as the fourth of the Seven Days Battles (Peninsula Campaign) of the Civil War. The main body of the Union Army of the Potomac had begun a general withdrawal toward the James River when. Confederate Brigadier General John B. Magruder, pursuing along the Richmond and York River Railroad and the Williamsburg Road, struck the rear guard of Union Major General Edwin Vose Sumner's II Corps with three brigades near Savage's Station while forces under Major General Thomas J. 'Stonewall" Jackson's divisions were stalled north of the Chickahominy River. Union forces continued to withdraw across White Oak Swamp, abandoning supplies and more than 2,500 wounded soldiers in a field hospital.

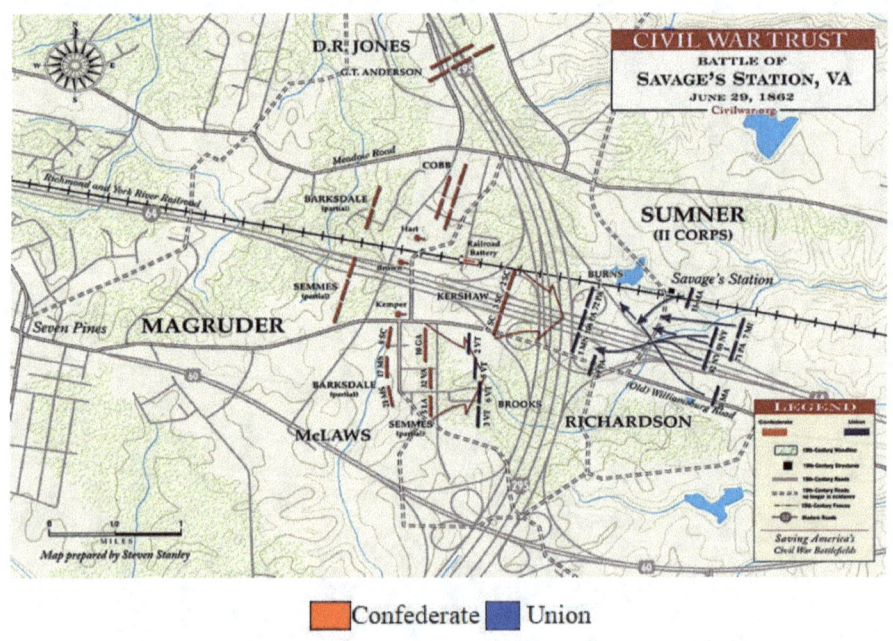

12-1: The Battle of Savage's Station

The wounded union soldiers were evacuated as rapidly as possible on railroad flatcars operated by the Richmond and York River Railroad. Some had makeshift awnings to protect them against the sun. They arrived at White House Landing on the Pamunkey River for transport by hospital ships to general hospitals in Washington, D.C. and other locations.

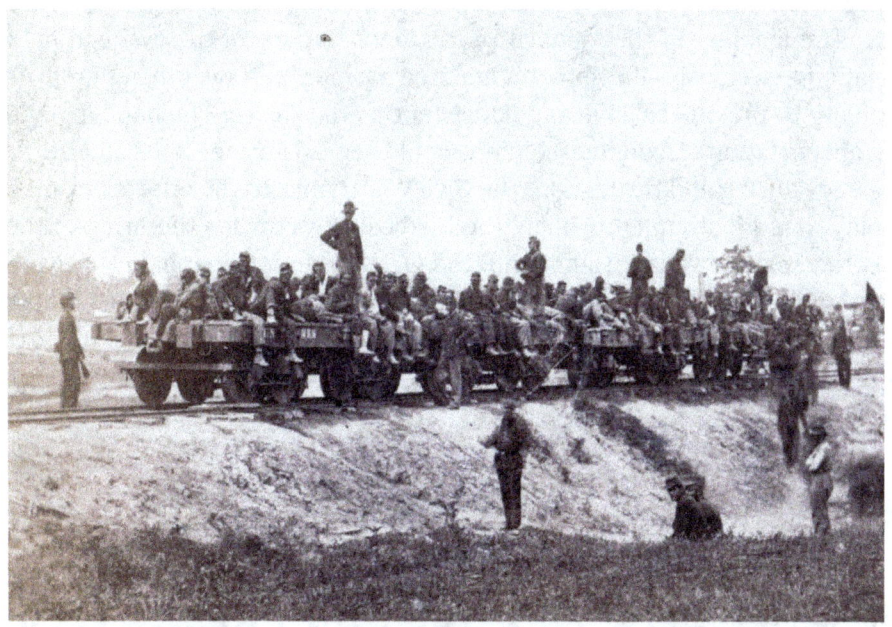

12-2: Wounded at Savage's Station

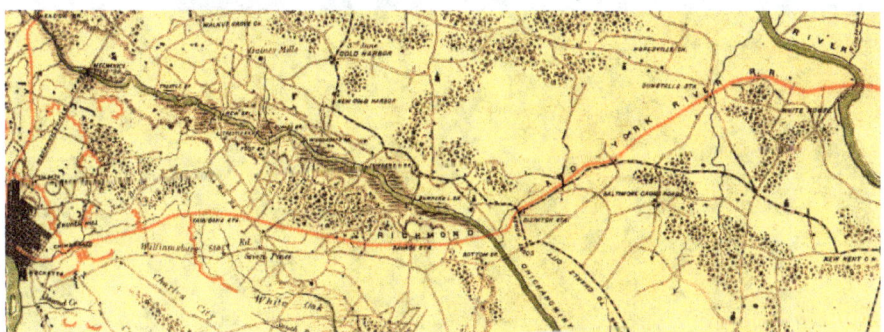

12-3: York River

CHAPTER 13
Doctor Letterman

The inability of the Medical Department to control the evacuation of patients seriously and in a regimented fashion seriously hampered its ability to provide reliable and consistent medical care. The handling and transportation of wounded soldiers would be transformed and gained efficiency during and throughout the Civil War thanks to the efforts of Union Major Dr. Jonathan Letterman, the Medical Director for the Army of the Potomac and William Hammond, the U.S. Surgeon General. Letterman's groundbreaking approach to the evacuation of wounded soldiers would earn him the title of "The Father of Modern Battlefield Medicine."

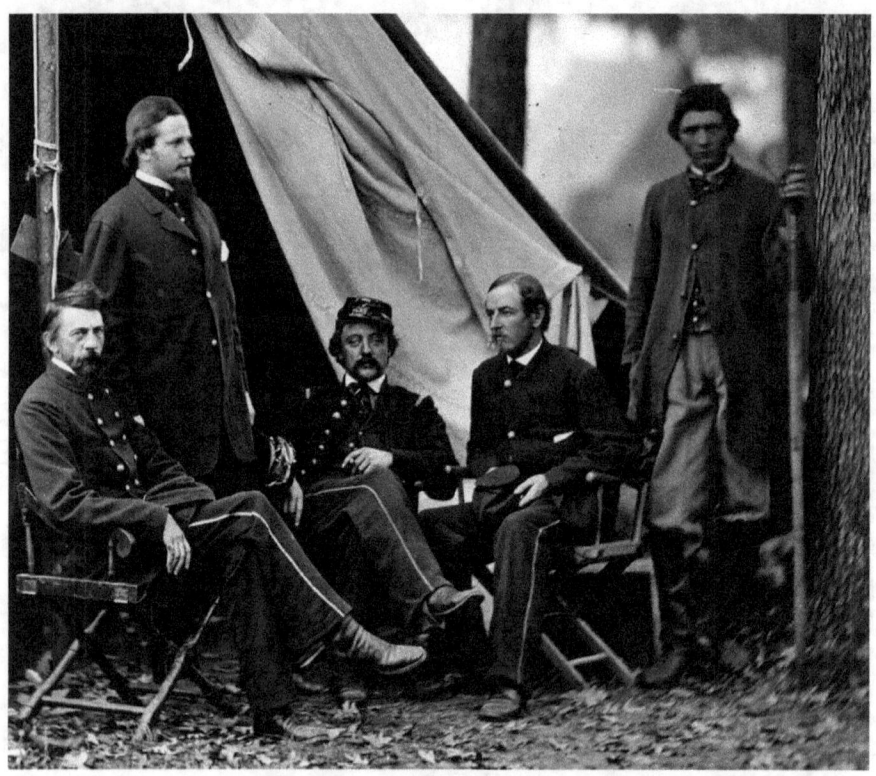

13-1: Photograph taken by Alexander Gardner, showing Dr. Letterman, sitting in front of the flag post, along with his staff.

Letterman and his staff further developed the U.S. Ambulance Corps based on a concept originated earlier by Charles S. Tripler, the former Medical Director. The so-called "Letterman Plan" involved the concept by which the ambulances of a division moved together with two stretcher-bearers and one driver per ambulance to move wounded from the field to dressing stations, and then on to the field hospital. This plan was implemented in August 1862 when McClellan issued General Orders No. 147 creating the Ambulance Corps for the Army of the Potomac. The Letterman Plan would get its trial by fire on September 17, 1862 at the Battle of Antietam.

CHAPTER 14
The Battle of Antietam

The Battle of Antietam, known as the Battle of Sharpsburg by the Confederacy, was fought on September 17, 1862, between the forces of Confederate General Robert E. Lee's Army of Northern Virginia and Union General George B. McClellan's Army of the Potomac located near Sharpsburg, Maryland and Antietam Creek. The battle proved to be the bloodiest day in United States history with a combined total of 22,717 dead, wounded, or missing. Lee withdrew from the battlefield first which is considered to be the technical definition of the tactical loser in a Civil War battle. Although many military historians considered the battle to be a draw, Antietam is considered as an initial turning point of the war and a victory for the Union because it ended Lee's strategic campaign (his first invasion of Union territory). The results of Antietam also allowed President Abraham Lincoln to issue the preliminary Emancipation Proclamation on September 22, which gave Confederate states until January 1, 1863, to return or else lose their slaves.

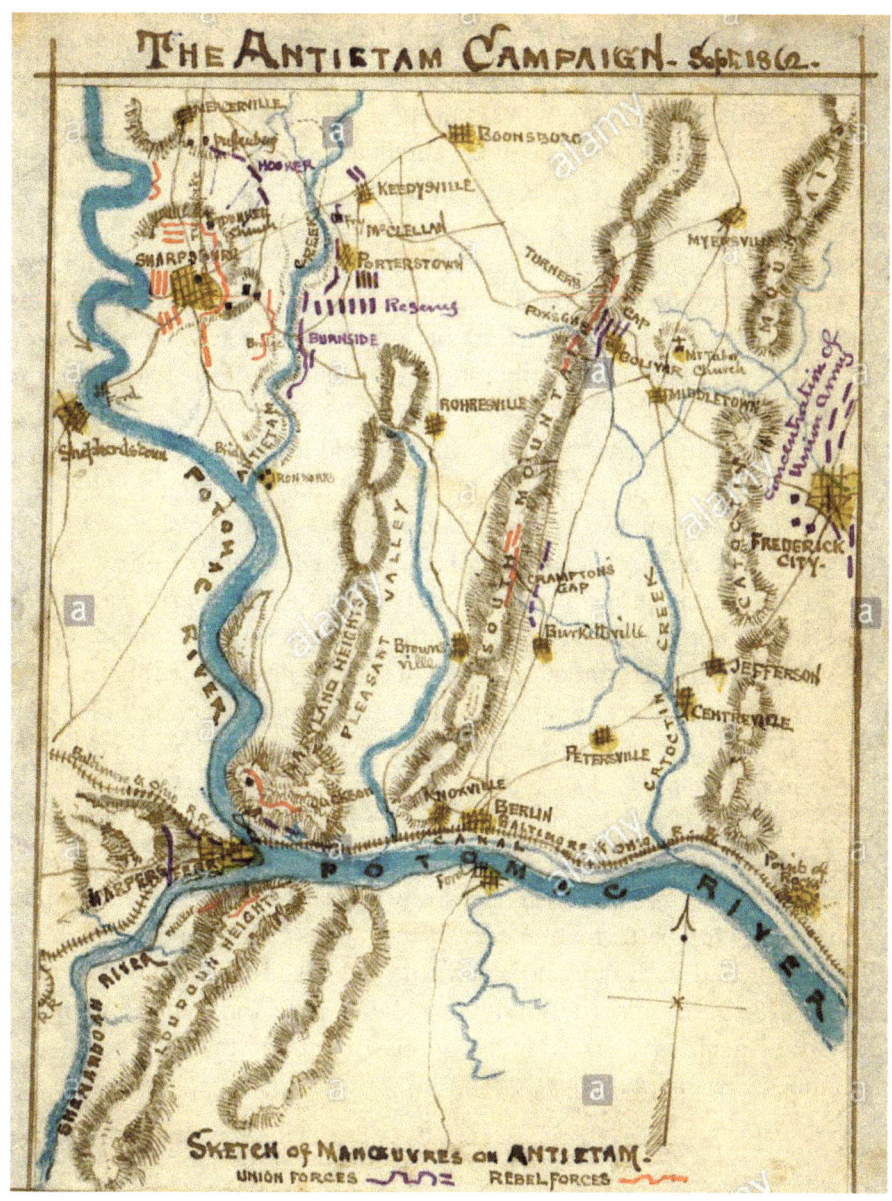

14-1: *The Battle of Antietem*

Despite the nearly 9,420 Union soldiers wounded during the battle, the heaviest casualties for a single day during the war, the ambulance corps had all of the wounded removed from the battlefield and under shelter by the evening of September 17th. Within three days, the wounded had been moved by horse-drawn ambulance to Frederick, Maryland. Every available space was put to use to accommodate the wounded and hospitals were established in churches, warehouses, hotels and private houses. Once these wounded were deemed "medically stabilized," they would be brought by ambulance wagon to the railroad terminal for evacuation to general hospitals.

Railroads were then used to remove the wounded from Frederick. Dr. Lettermen attempted to coordinate the arrival of battlefield ambulances with the train schedule posted at the Frederick depot. Letterman later recalled the difficulty in coordinating the movement of the patients:

> "It was imperative that the trains should leave at the proper hours, no one interfering with another; that they should halt at Middletown, where food and rest, with such surgical aid as might be required, could be given at this village at the proper time for the proper number; that the hospitals in Frederick should not be over crowded, and the ambulances should arrive at the railroad depot at the required time to meet the Baltimore trains. With rare exceptions this was accomplished, and all the wounded, whose lives would not be jeopardized, were sent carefully away."

The wounded were most likely loaded into converted freight or boxcars with the floors lined with hay, straw or blankets in order to cushion the ride. Doctor Letterman observed that "The capacious barns, abundantly provided with hay and straw, the delightful weather with which we were favored, and the kindness exhibited by the people, afforded increased facilities to the medical department for taking care of the wounded thrown upon it by that battle."

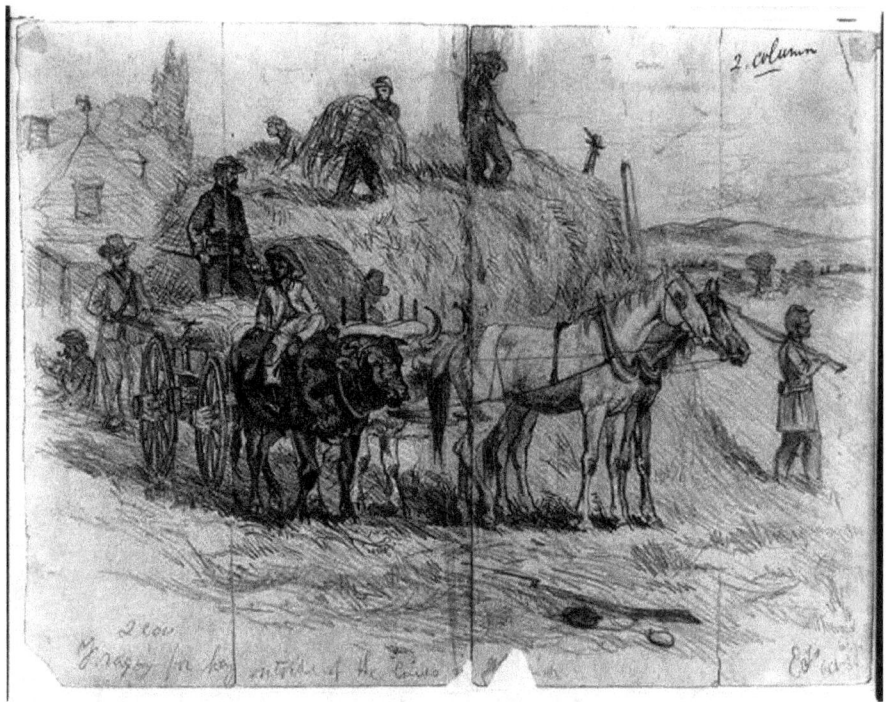

14-2: Foraging for hay.

Openings or slots were made in the cars in order to allow fresh air to flow in.

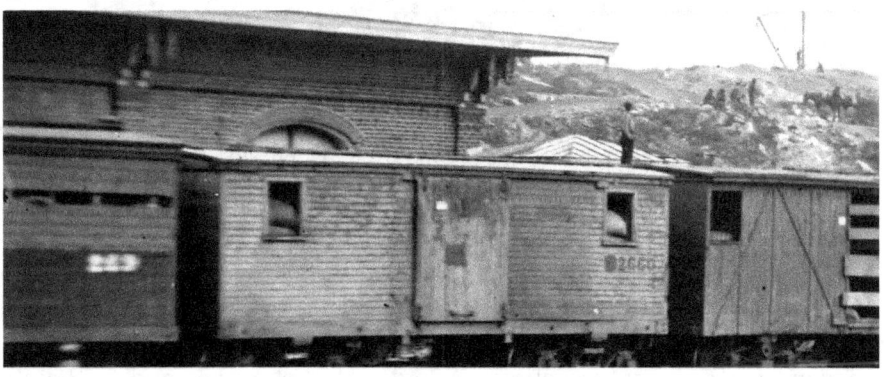

14-3: Civil War box cars from film.

According to Doctor Letterman, of the approximately 9,400 soldiers wounded, only 5,000 remained in Frederick a month and a half after the battle, reducing the burden on a town with an approximate civilian population of 8,000. The dispersal of the sick and wounded to hospitals that could be supported by larger cities improved the quality of care available to the patient and allowed the surgeons in Frederick to concentrate their efforts on the more seriously wounded cases that remained.

Records from the Frederick Office of Medical Department of Transportation showed that 6,362 wounded soldiers, from the Battle of Antietam, were quickly removed from Frederick via the Baltimore and Ohio Railroad, on special trains, including 1,356 of these going to Baltimore city, 3,329 sent to Washington, D.C., and 1,677 to Philadelphia. The image of the Baltimore and Ohio Railroad system was obtained from the *New York Herald*, Sunday, September 7, 1862.

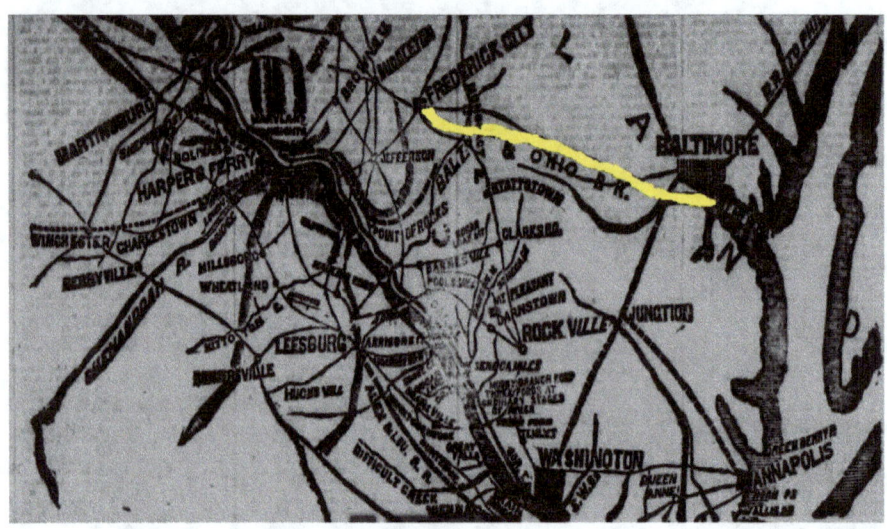

14-4: Baltimore & Ohio (B & O) Railroad

This following image shows the arrival of President Lincoln for a visit to Frederick, Maryland on October 4, 1862. His special train has arrived at the Baltimore and Ohio Railroad terminal, on South Market Street, which is the structure to the right with the large American flag proudly on display. At the intersection of South Market Street and All Saints Street, President Abraham Lincoln spoke from a railroad car platform to Frederick residents assembled in the street on October 4, 1862. He was in town to view the battlefields of South Mountain and Antietam and to call on General George L. Hartsuff who was recuperating here from a wound suffered at Antietam.

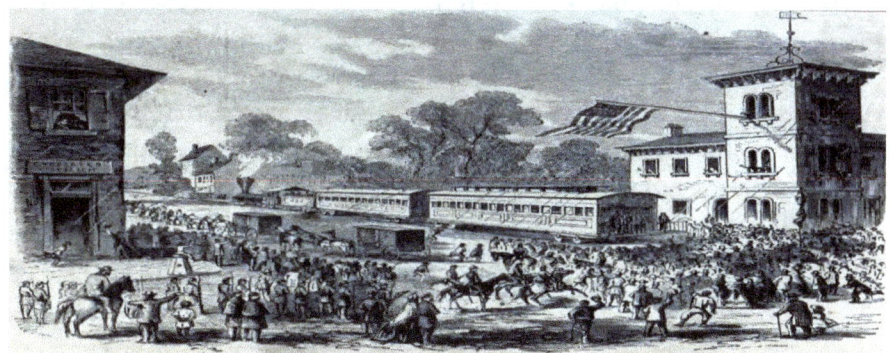

14-5: President Lincoln arrives in Frederick, Maryland

According to the book entitled *One Vast Hospital* by Terry Reimer, large numbers of wounded soldiers were sent from the battlefield hospitals, through Frederick, to military hospitals in other cities as soon as the railroad bridge over the Monocacy River was reopened on September 21. General Lee had decided to move his army out of war-torn Virginia, and on September 4, 1862, he led more than 40,000 Confederate troops across the Potomac at White's Ford to Frederick. Shortly after that, Confederate troops destroyed B&O Railroad bridges over the Potomac and Monocacy Rivers, as well as other railroad property in the region. Because of the loss of these bridges, the medical supplies on hand in Frederick were limited to what they had before the battle.

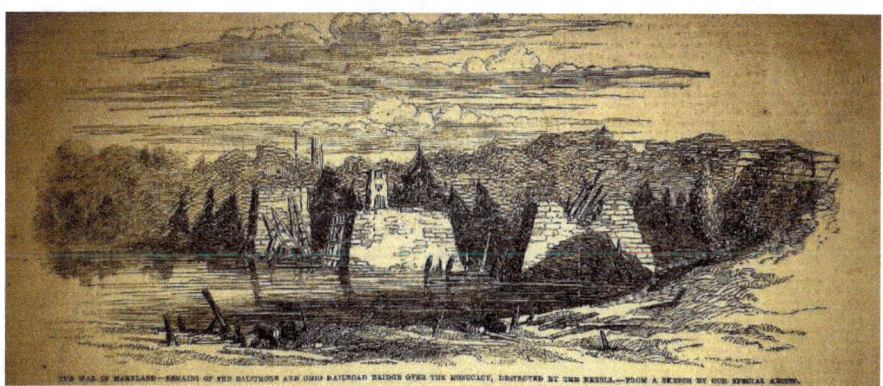

14-6: Monocacy Bridge

In a real sense, Frederick served as an evacuation hospital moving men out as expetiously as possible. Most of the wounded were sent to General Hospitals in Philadelphia, Washington, D.C. and Baltimore, and some were sent to an extensive convalescent camp in Alexandria, Virginia. Twenty-two ambulances were required just to transport the wounded from the Frederick hospitals to the trains. One surgeon noted that 1,200 were transferred in one train of cars. Many of these wounded men remained in Frederick for a day or so. Most of these men were he less seriously wounded and were give a night's rest in Frederick before being sent on to other hospitals. Many of these men probably stayed the night at the U.S. Hotel which is adjacent to the B&O Railroad Terminal.

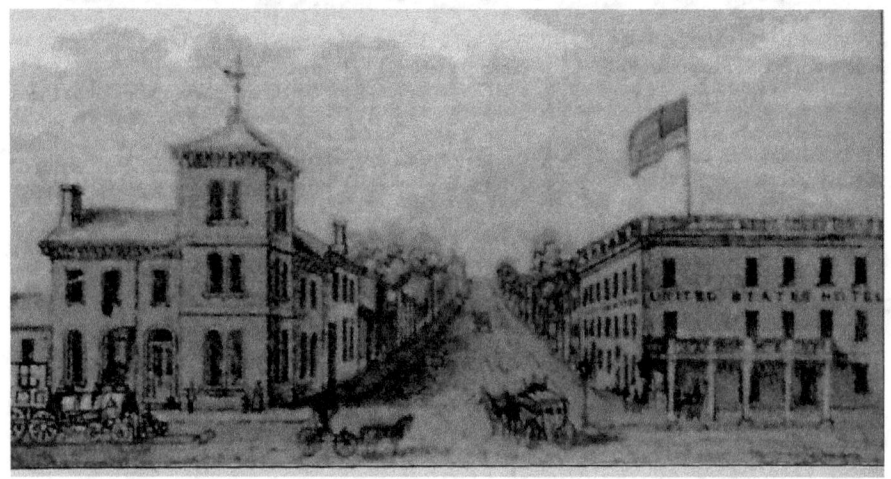

14-7: This 1854 drawing from View of Frederick, Maryland shows the U.S. Hotel on the right (west) and the train station on the left (east). View is looking south on South Market Street.

CHAPTER 15
The Battle of Fredericksburg

The Battle of Fredericksburg, December 11-14, 1862, was perhaps the Confederacy's most lopsided victory of the Civil War. Union Major General Ambrose E. Burnside, leading the Army of the Potomac, charged with aggressively pursuing and destroying General Robert E. Lee's Army of Northern Virginia, instead led his own Army of the Potomac to what was perhaps its greatest defeat. On December 13, Burnside sent six Union divisions across an open field against Lee's well-fortified line, causing such slaughter that Burnside wept openly at the outcome and Lee was inspired to utter his famous remark to his subordinates, "It is well that war is so terrible. We should grow too fond of it."

The Fredericksburg defeat was one of the lowest points for Union fortunes in the war. The Union Army suffered 1,180 killed and 9,028 wounded about twice as many as the Confederacy suffered. The Union Army was forced to evacuate 1,500 of their wounded via the Richmond, Fredericksburg and Potomac Railroad's Falmouth Station to its rail facilities at Acquia Creek where these wounded were evacuated by hospital ships belonging to the Potomac Steamboat Company and other sponsors to general hospitals in Washington, D.C. The Confederates abandoned the site in 1862 and destroyed the railroad and wharves. The Union moved in and rebuilt the facilities, but destroyed them again when they evacuated the area in September 1862. In November 1862, the Union army under General Burnside rebuilt Acquia Landing yet again to use as a supply depot for the Fredericksburg campaign. When they left in June 1863 to march to Gettysburg, this time the Confederates destroyed it. The Union rebuilt it in May 1864, but abandoned it for supply bases further south. The Confederates destroyed it again and this time, it was not rebuilt. Acquia Landing had also been used to move troops as well as supplies.

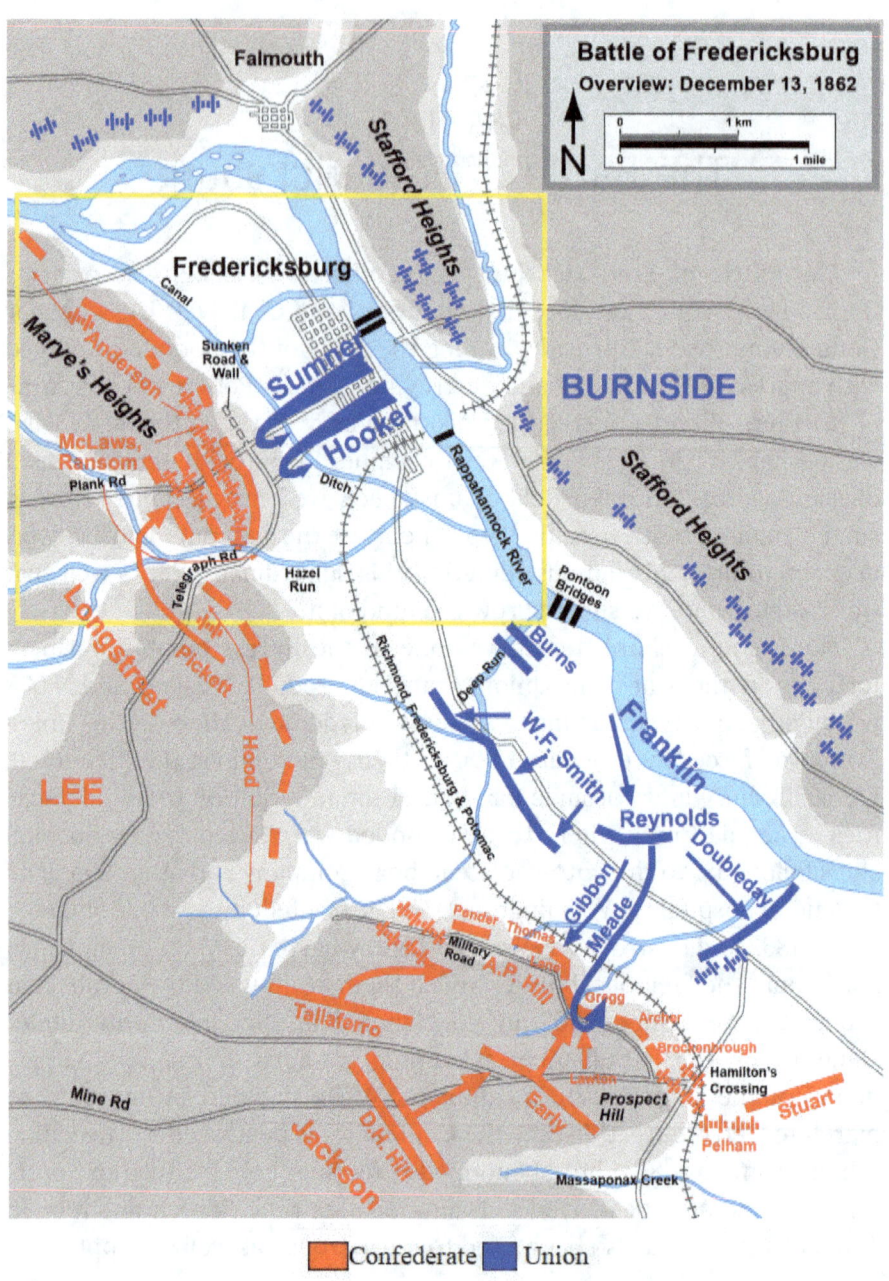

15-1: The Battle of Fredericksburg

The Battle of Fredericksburg | 97

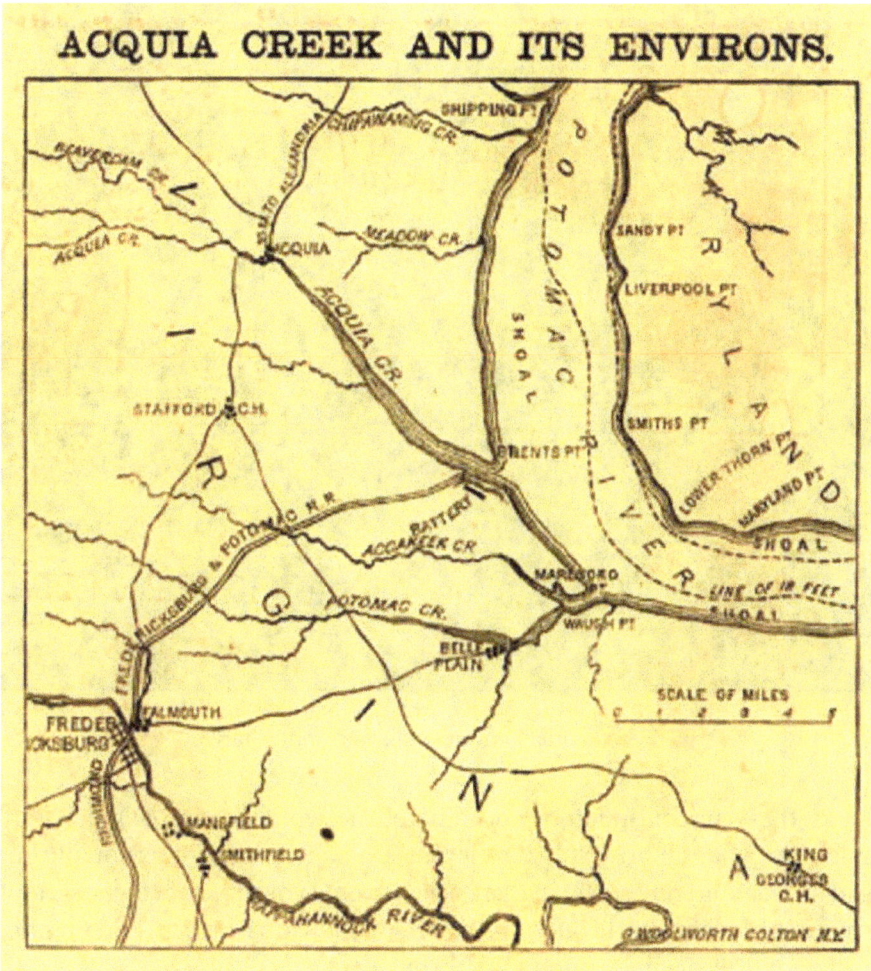

15-2: Acquia Creek

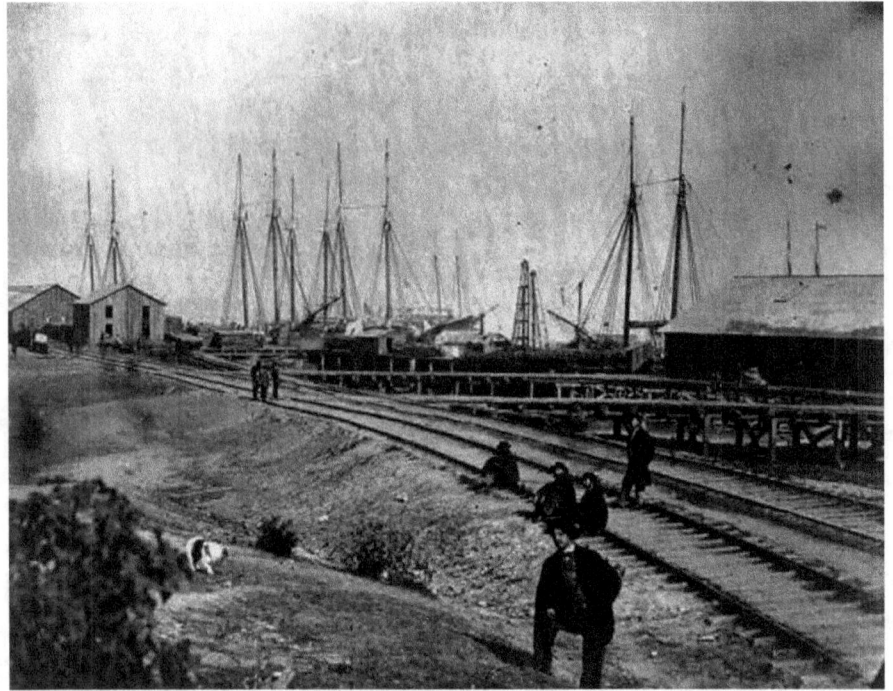

15-3: Acquia Landing, Railroad and Wharf

As the war continued, a coordinated network of railroads, hospital ships and general hospitals developed. Unlike the carefully thought out and implemented Letterman Plan, this system evolved on its own without any central planning through the efforts of individual civilian and military surgeons, railroad men and philanthropists.

The Medical Department of the Army of the Potomac had been organized according to the Letterman Plan when General Ambrose Burnside attacked Fredericksburg on December 13, 1862. Since Letterman had planned to treat the wounded near the battle at a hospital in Falmouth, Virginia, he had not made preparations for moving them out of the combat zone. When Burnside ordered the evacuation of all of the wounded to Washington, Letterman objected arguing that his patients could not withstand a winter rail journey. Burnside, desiring to resume the offensive, was adamant and Letterman was compelled to order the evacuation.

Assistant Surgeon DeWitt Peters, who had been detailed by Letterman to convey 1,500 wounded soldiers to Washington, D.C., described the journey, "The transportation from Falmouth to Acquia Creek was ample, but many of the cars consisted of simple platforms without covering, and were ill adapted for transporting men badly wounded, especially in midwinter; and, for this reason, some of the unfortunate suffered much. Many of them had lost their blankets, but at the depot I found a supply belonging to the Sanitary Commission, and these I appropriated. There was no straw in the cars for making beds and none on hand that I could take for the purpose. At Acquia Creek, we transferred to hospital ships. Here again, there was ample room for the men, but nothing was provided for them to rest upon save hard boards of decks. We were well supplied with rations, nurses and attendants, who did everything possible to make the wounded comfortable. ...The time occupied in making the journey to Washington was seventeen hours." Despite the arduous journey and the cold weather, approximately 6,000 wounded were evacuated without any fatalities. Although Letterman was criticized for sending the wounded in open railcars in the middle of winter, the cold weather probably saved lives by contracting blood vessels and minimizing hemorrhaging.

While the Fredericksburg campaign turned into a tactical debacle, the medical efforts were successful and became a model for how the wounded would be handled in the future. The Letterman Plan was proven as an effective strategy for handling casualties. The sudden order to move the wounded out of Falmouth to make room for additional casualties from an anticipated future combat was a common feature in future campaigns. The trip from Fredericksburg to Washington, although extremely uncomfortable for the patients, proved that the wounded could survive such a journey, even under adverse conditions. The Fredericksburg campaign proved the need for specialized hospital trains to evacuate the wounded.

CHAPTER 16
The Chancellorsville Campaign

The Chancellorsville Campaign was fought from April 30 to May 6, 1863, in Spotsylvania County, Virginia, which culminated in the Battle of Chancellorsville on May 4-6. Two related battles were fought nearby on May 3 in the vicinity of Fredericksburg. The campaign pitted Union Army Major General Joseph Hooker's Army of the Potomac against an army less than half its size, the Confederate Army of Northern Virginia under the leadership of General Robert E. Lee. The combined Union forces totaled 13,868 soldiers while the South fielded only 60,298 men.

Chancellorsville is known as Lee's "perfect battle," by military historians, because of his risky decision to divide his army in the presence of a much larger enemy force resulted in a significant Confederate victory. The victory, a product of Lee's audacity and Hooker's timid decision-making, was tempered by heavy casualties, including the irreplaceable loss of Lieutenant General Thomas J. "Stonewall" Jackson. Jackson was hit by friendly fire which required his left arm to be amputated. He died of pneumonia eight days later, a loss that Lee likened to losing his right arm. Lee's difficulty in replacing the large number of men he lost in battle contributed to his inability to prevent the Union successful withdrawal from the battlefield. Although Chancellorsville was considered to be a Confederate victory, although a Pyrrhic one, the terrible loss of Jackson considerably lessened its overall success for the South. During the Chancellorsville campaign, 1,606 Union soldiers were killed and 9,762 men wounded while the South had 1,665 men killed and 9,061 wounded.

The Chancellorsville Campaign | 101

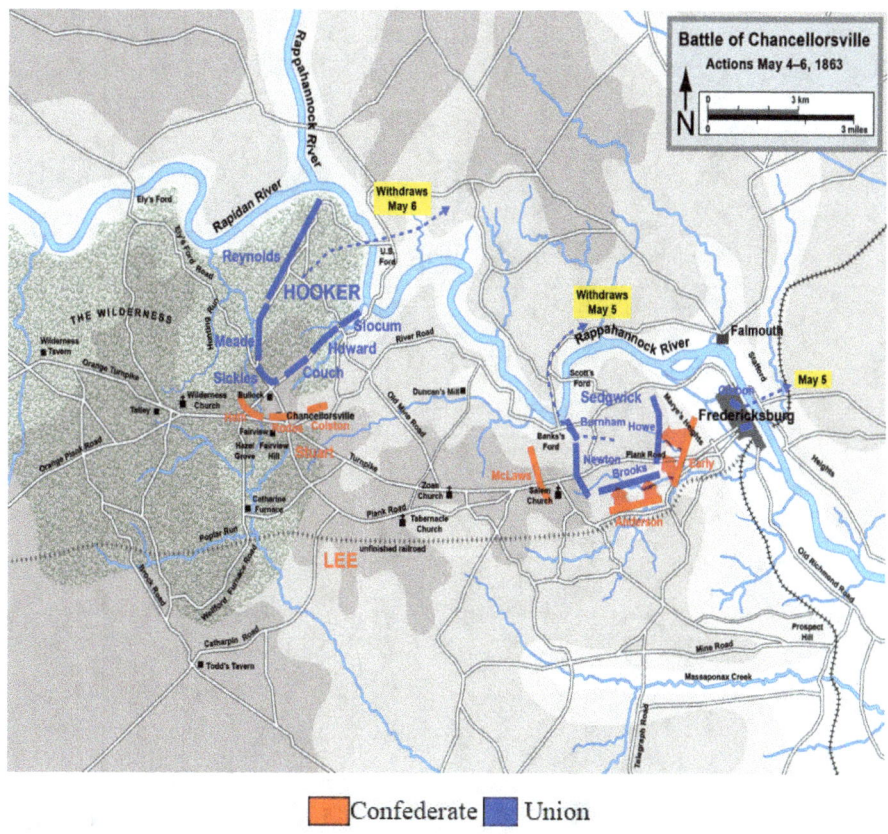

16-1: Union withdrawal of troops from the field during the last days of the Battle of Chancellorsville.

The Richmond, Fredericksburg, and Potomac Railroad Bridge over the Rappahannock River at Fredericksburg was destroyed and rebuilt several times during the Civil War.

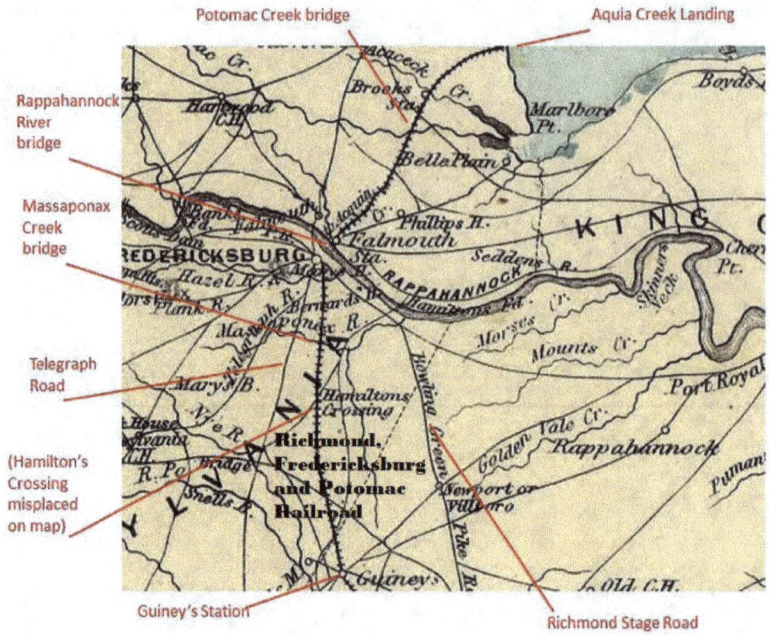

16-2: Chancellorsville Campaign

During the Chancellorsville campaign, it was destroyed by Confederate batteries situated on Marye's Heights overlooking Fredericksburg across the Rappahannock River. The destruction of this key bridge prevented the railroad from moving the wounded Union soldiers from its Falmouth Station in Fredericksburg to the Aquia Creek Landing.

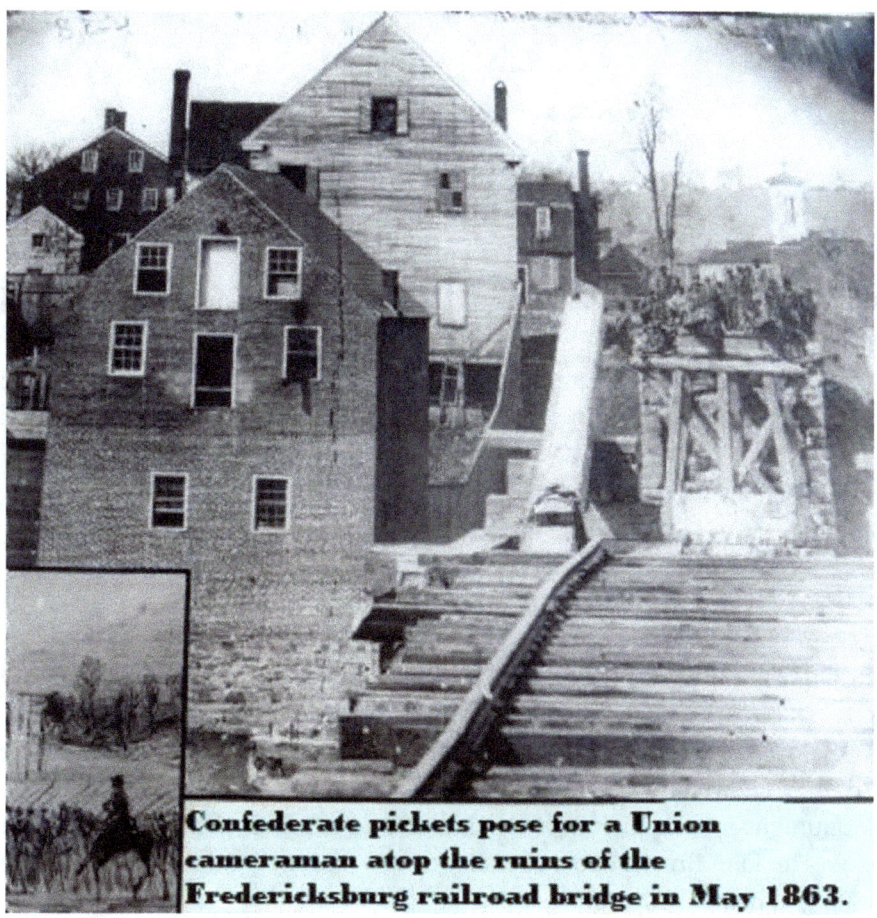

16-3: Fredericksburg Railroad Bridge

With the bridge gone, the wounded were instead loaded onto Federal ambulance wagons. This loading was reportedly slow and tedious; half of the wounded couldn't help themselves in anyway. Four badly wounded soldiers were placed on the floor of each wagon side by side; those who could sit up were closely packed on the seats.

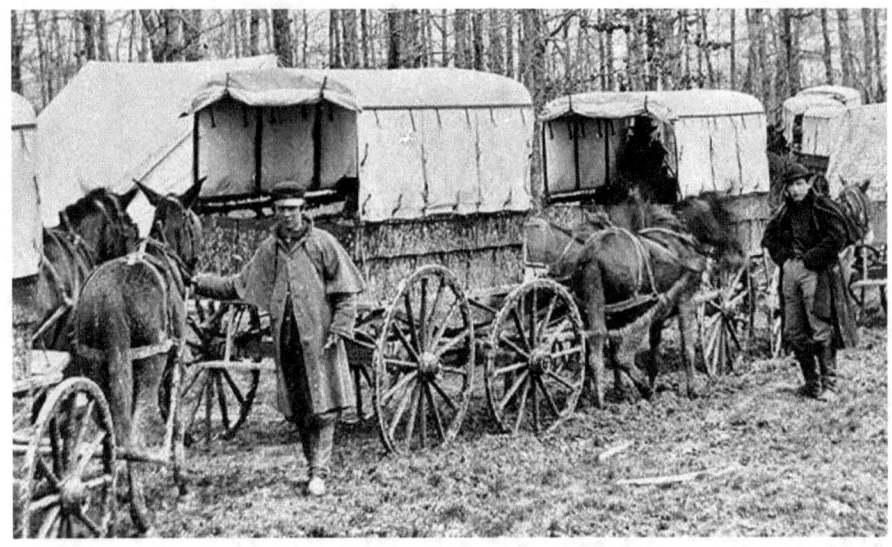

16-4: Ambulances

Once at Aquia Creek Landing, these wounded were transferred to hospital ships for their trip up the Potomac River to Washington, D.C.

Below, the hospital ship *John Brooks* is seen passing in front of the Sixth Street Wharf in Washington, D.C. note the unfinished Washington Monument in the far left of the image and the U.S. Capital in the right side. The *John Brooks* had a capacity of 400 patients and saw action in the 1862 Peninsula campaign.

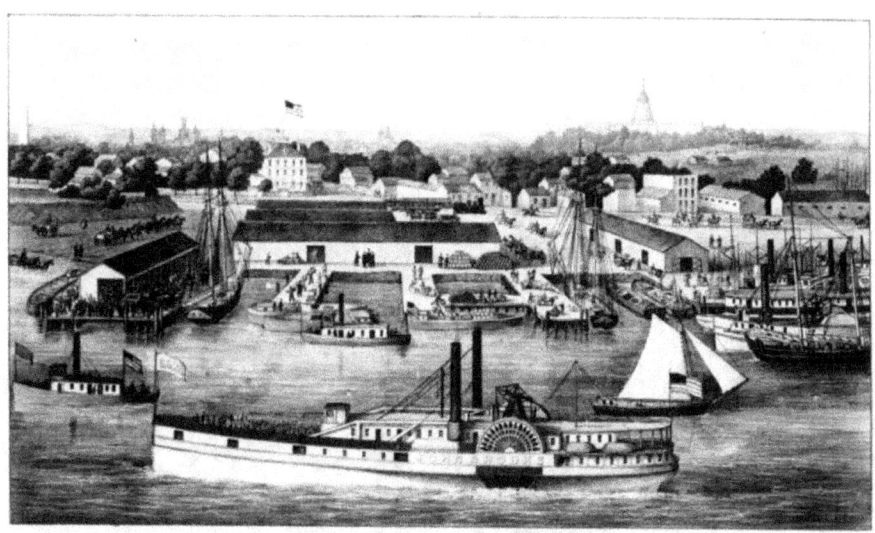

16-5: Hospital Transport Ship *John Brooks* passing the Sixth Street Wharf in Washington, DC

During the war, Washington's busy wharves, notably the Sixth Street Wharf, were the focal point for moving people and supplies into and out of the city. Here the wounded from the Virginia battlefields were off-loaded from steamboats to await transport to the city's many hospitals. The most severe cases were taken to the nearest – Armory Square Hospital—about ten blocks north on Seventh Street where it crossed the National Mall.

The noted poet Walt Whitman was a nurse during the Civil War and published an account of his war experiences in *Memoranda During the War*.

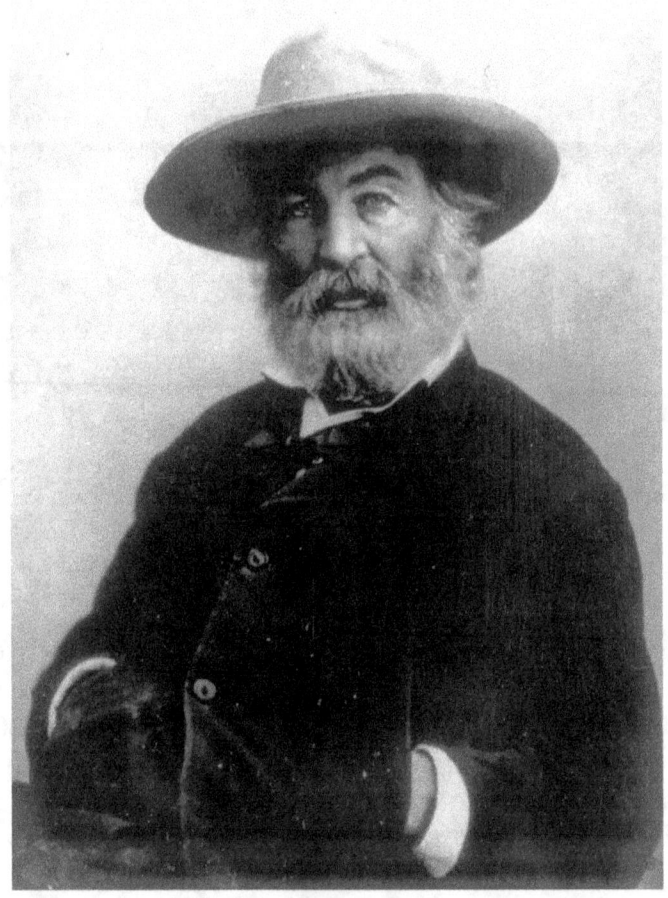

16-6: Walt Whitman

Of Washington's many hospitals, Whitman visited Armory Square most often, as he explained in a letter to his mother. "I devote myself much to Armory Square Hospital because it contains by far the worst cases, most repulsive wounds, has the most suffering & most need of consolation go every day without fail, & often at night sometimes stay very late no one interferes with me, guards, doctors, nurses, nor any one am let to take my own course."

One of six model hospitals constructed in 1862, Armory Square took its name from the Old Armory on the Mall, around which the hospital was built. Its location (the current site of the National Air and Space Museum) placed it nearest the steamboat landing at the foot of Seventh Street, S.W., and near the tracks of the Washington and Alexandria Railroad, which ran along Maryland Avenue. As a result, Armory Square received the most serious casualties from the Virginia battlefields, those too ill to travel any farther. From August 1861 to January 1865, Armory Square recorded the largest number of deaths of any Washington military hospital, 1,339 out of 18,291 deaths.

Here is his account of his experiences following the Battle of Chancellorsville while serving at the hospital.

> *Wounded from Chancellorsville, May, '63.*
> *As I write this, the wounded have begun to arrive from Hooker's command from bloody Chancellorsville. I was down among the first arrivals. The men in charge of them told me the bad cases were yet to come. If that is so I pity them, for these are bad enough. You ought to see the scene of the wounded arriving at the landing here foot of Sixth street, at night. Two boat loads came about half-past seven last night. little after eight it rain'd a long and violent shower. The poor, pale, helpless soldiers had been debark'd, and lay around on the wharf and neighborhood anywhere. The rain was, probably, grateful to them; at any rate they were exposed to it. The few torches light up the spectacle. All around -- on the wharf, on the ground, out on side places -- the men are lying on blankets, old quilts, &c., with bloody rags bound round heads, arms, and legs. The attendants are few, and at night few outsiders also -- only a few hard-work'd transportation men and drivers. (The wounded are getting to be common, and people grow callous.) The men, whatever their condition, lie there, and patiently wait till their turn comes to be taken up. Near by, the ambulances are now arriving clusters, and one after another is call'd to back up and take its load. Extreme cases are sent off on stretehers. The men generally make little or no ado, whatever their sufferings. A few groans that cannot be suppress'd, and occasionally a scream of pain as they lift a man into the ambulance... Today, as I write, hundreds more are expected, and to-morrow and the next day more, and so on for many days. Quite often they arrive at the rate of 1000 a day.*

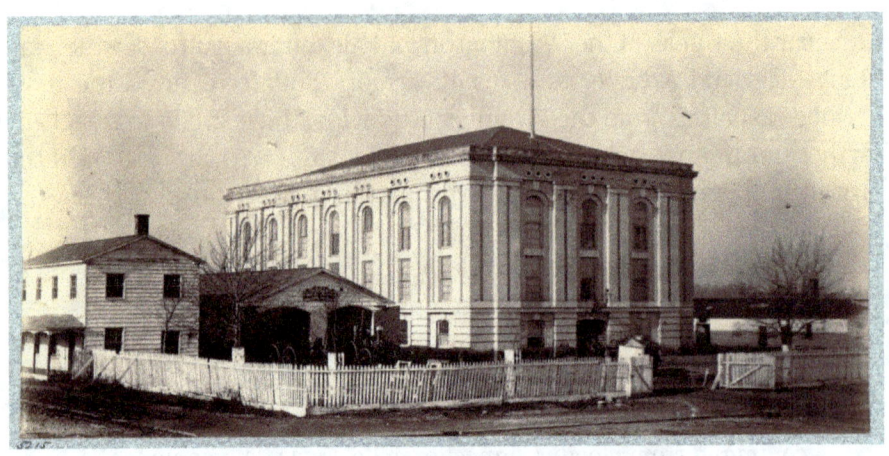

16-7: Armory Square Hospital in Washington, D.C. during the Civil War.

The following image shows convalescents posing for the camera in Ward K of the Armory Square Hospital. The hospital had 1,000 beds and was one of the largest such general hospitals, located in the Nation's Capital, caring for wounded soldiers.

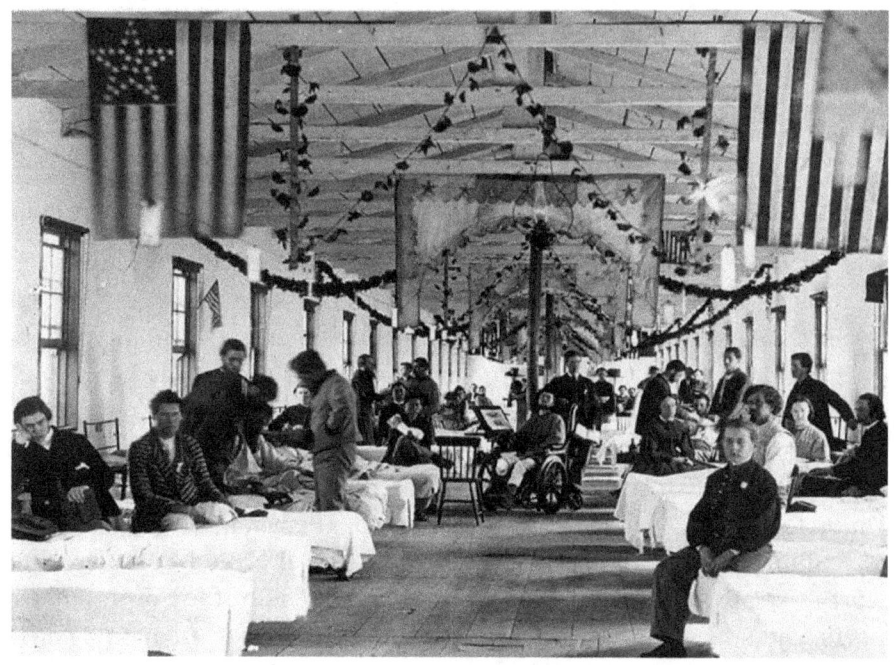

16-8: Convalescents in Ward K of Armory Square Hospital.

"Thus in silence in dreams' projections,
Returning, resuming, I thread my way through the hospitals,
The hurt and wounded I pacify with soothing hand,
I sit by the restless all the dark night, some are so young,
Some suffer so much, I recall the experience sweet and sad,
Many a soldier's loving arms about this neck have cross'd and rested,
Many a soldier's kiss dwells on these bearded lips."
-- Wound Dressing, by Walt Whitman

CHAPTER 17
The Vicksburg Campaign

The Vicksburg Campaign and eventual siege was conducted during the months of April-July 1863. In a series of maneuvers, Union Major General Ulysses S. Grant and his Army of the Tennessee crossed the Mississippi River and drove the Confederate Army of Mississippi, led by Lieutenant General John C. Pemberton, into the defensive lines surrounding the fortress city of Vicksburg, Mississippi.

Following the loss of Island No. 10 on the upper Mississippi River to Union forces, on April 8, 1862, Vicksburg was the last major Confederate stronghold on the river; therefore, capturing it would complete the North's strategy of blocking all commercial traffic to the South's major ports, the so-called Anaconda Plan. When two major assaults against the Confederate fortifications, on May 19 and 22, were repulsed with heavy casualties, Grant decided to besiege the city beginning on May 25. After holding out for more than forty days, with their supplies nearly gone, the garrison surrendered on July 4. The successful ending of the Vicksburg campaign significantly degraded the ability of the Confederacy to maintain its war effort. This action, combined with the surrender of Port Hudson to Major General Nathaniel P. Banks on July 9, yielded command of the Mississippi River to the Union forces, who would hold it for the rest of the war.

The Confederate surrender on July 4, when combined with General Robert E. Lee's defeat at Gettysburg by Major General George Meade the previous day, is considered, by many military historians, to be the turning point of the entire war. It effectively cut off the Trans-Mississippi Theatre (containing the states of Arkansas, Texas and part of Louisiana) from the rest of the Confederate States, effectively splitting the Confederacy in two for the duration of the war.

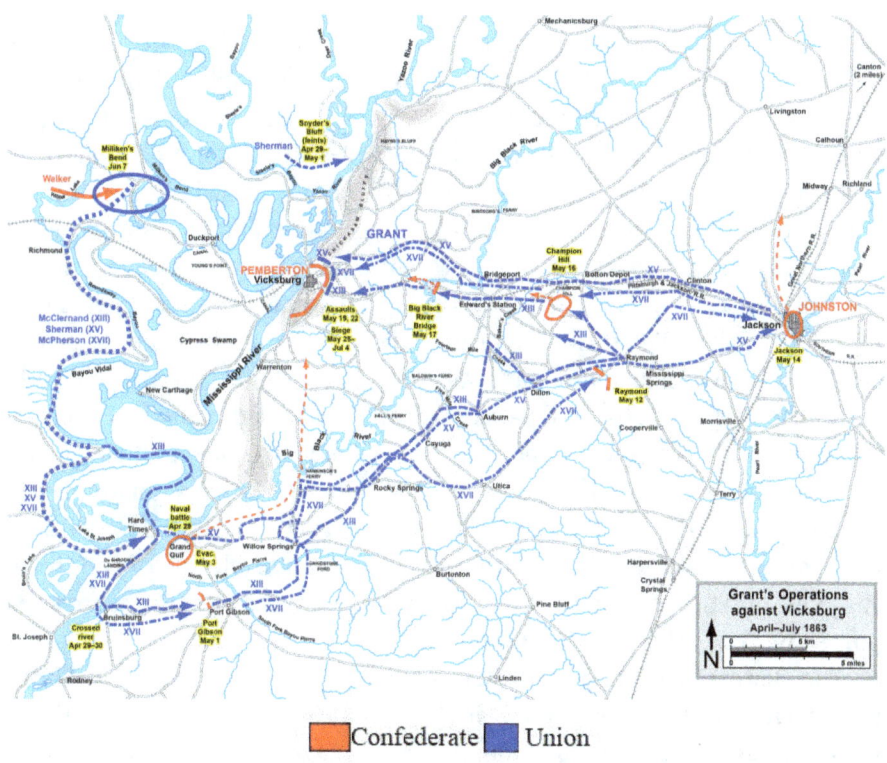

17-1: The Vicksburg Campaign

The Vicksburg Campaign resulted in 3,793 wounded Union soldiers. In addition, Grant's troops experienced a high degree of sickness due to widespread cases of malaria caused by the extremely hot and swampy terrain in which they had to fight.

The hospital ship USS *Red Rover* would play an instrumental and pivotal role in the handling and evacuation of these wounded during the entire Vicksburg Campaign. It was undoubtedly the most famous steamer to serve as a hospital ship in the waters of the Mississippi River during the Civil War. Neither the Union nor Confederacy had ever created a complete hospital aboard a steamship before, nor *Red Rover* was refitted with innovations never before found on a ship, all designed to help the sick and wounded. Rooms at the back of the ship had open walls to allow for better air circulation, and patients who had contagious diseases were put in these, as well as on several separate floating barges attached to the back of the ship. This helped keep the spread of very contagious diseases, such as measles and typhus, from infecting everyone on board. *Red Rover* also carried enough medical and food supplies for two hundred patients and the entire crew for up to three months—everything the hospital staff needed was on board, making the ship completely self-sufficient if it needed to be.

Caring for the sick and wounded became so overwhelming, due to superb care afforded by the ship, that fleet commander Charles Henry Davis had to issue an order to limit the number of patients being sent to the ship—it seemed like every sick or injured soldier wanted to be cared for on *Red Rover*. The order apparently didn't work all the time, since the ship's log shows that many patients came on without papers, or simply under the verbal approval of particular doctors or high-ranking officials.

During the war, the captured side-wheel steamer named by its Confederate owner the *Red Rover*, proved to be the U.S. Navy's first complete hospital ship. The first vessel thus designated as a Navy hospital ship had a crew of twelve officers and thirty-five men, exclusive of the thirty surgeons and nurses aboard. **The mostly male nurses onboard were supported by the Sisters of the Holly Cross.**

The Sisters' duties, particularly when serving on the floating hospital boat USS *Red Rover*, **consisted of cleaning, laundering, administering medicine, nourishing the sick and providing "spiritual comfort for patients." The Sisters of the Holy Cross traveled on the Mississippi River aboard the** *Red Rover*, **collecting injured soldiers, caring for them aboard the ship and depositing them at hospitals in Memphis, Mound City and Cairo. The** *Red Rover* **attempted to reach Vicksburg, the "City of the Siege"; after witnessing a boat blockade and firing at Vicksburg, the Sisters helped "lift the bruised and broken soldiers from rivers of blood."**

Ann Stokes was first taken aboard a Union Naval vessel as "contraband" in 1863.

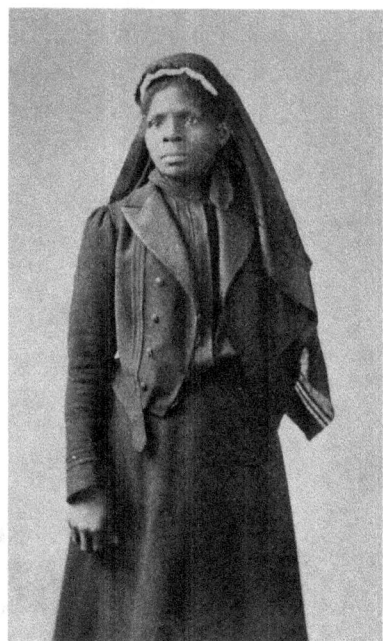

17-2: Ann Stokes

As was typical of most former slaves, Stokes could not read or write, but was hired as a nurse. She worked under the direction of the Sisters of the Holy Cross nuns aboard the USS *Red Rover*. **Although the "regular corps of nurses" on board the *Red Rover* consisted of males, Sister Angela of the Sisters of the Holy Cross offered the assistance of that order in providing nurses when needed.** The offer was gratefully accepted, and various Sisters served on board in a temporary capacity from time to time in 1862. Stokes became the first African American woman to serve on board a U.S. military vessel and was among the first women to serve as nurses in the Navy.

Black sailors constituted a significant segment of naval manpower and nearly doubled the number of black soldiers serving in the U.S. Army. They did manual labor or worked in general assistance, damage control units, and small arms crews, but their maritime skills were strategically important on the Mississippi River and in the work of the Mississippi Squadron. At the combined army and navy assault on Vicksburg, commanders took great advantage of the knowledge and experience of the black sailors. As the hospital ship assigned to the Mississippi Squadron, the USS *Red*

Rover sailed with them during actions. Thus, contrabands, both male and female, played an important role during the war, particularly on the USS *Red Rover*.

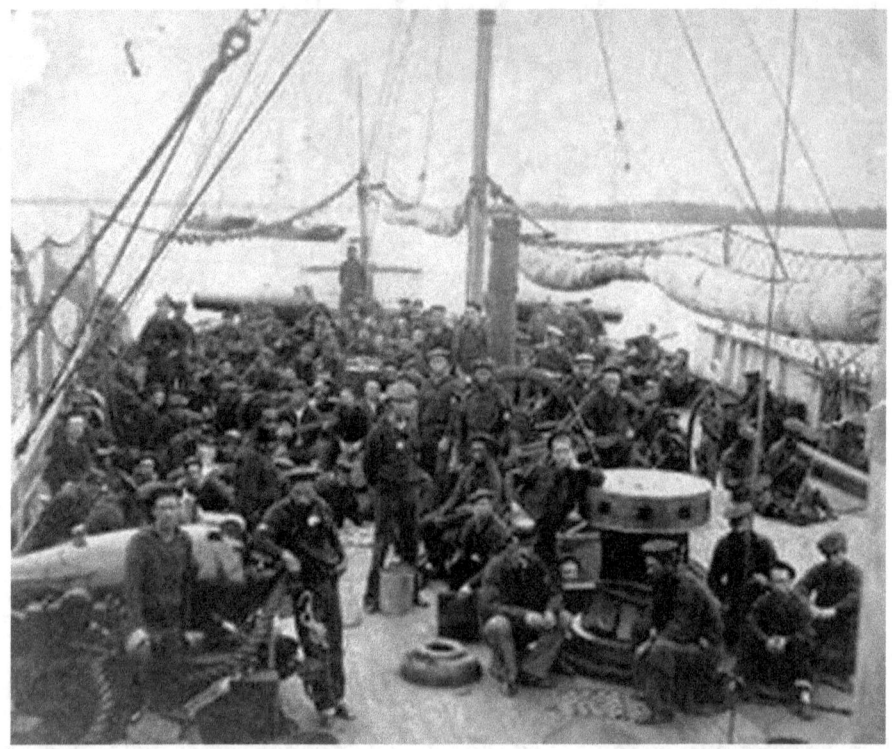

17-3: Hospital Transport Ship *Red Rover*

The 650-ton side-wheel steamer was built at Cape Girardeau, Missouri in 1859. It was originally used as living quarters for the men manning the Confederate States' Floating Battery New Orleans. When New Orleans was bombarded by the Union's Western Gunboat Flotilla in March 1862, the *Red Rover* was hit by a shell that pierced her top and slanted through all her decks to the bottom. Although she leaked considerably, the ship was in no danger of sinking. She was captured by the Union gunboat *Mound City* and almost immediately prepared as a floating hospital for the casualties of the North. Not long after her capture, the renamed USS *Red Rover* became a haven for many injured men and officers of the apprehending gunboat. That summer, the ship was renovated by the Army Quartermaster Corps to include laundries, bathroom facilities, elevators to upper decks, surgery and operating rooms, nine water closets, separate kitchens for crew and patients, and gauze blinds to keep out smoke and cinders from the convalescents' berth deck. Commander Captain Alexander M. Pennock reported to his Flag officer, "The boat is supplied with everything necessary for the restoration of health for the disabled seamen." From April 1863 to the fall of Vicksburg early in July, she cared for the sick and wounded of that campaign and supplemented her medical support of Union forces by provisioning other ships of the Mississippi Squadron with ice and fresh meat. She also provided burial details and sent medical personnel ashore when and where needed. The USS *Red Rover* continued her service along the river, taking on sick and wounded and delivering medicine and supplies until the fall of 1864. In October of that year, she began her last supply run. After delivering medical stores to ships at Helena and on the White, Red, and Yazoo Rivers, she transferred patients to Hospital Pinckney at Memphis, Tennessee and headed north. Arriving at Mound City, Illinois on December 11, she remained there, caring for Navy patients, until she was decommissioned on November 17, 1865. Having admitted 2,947 patients during her career, she transferred her last 11 to Grampus on that date. On November 29, she was sold at public auction to A. M. Carpenter.

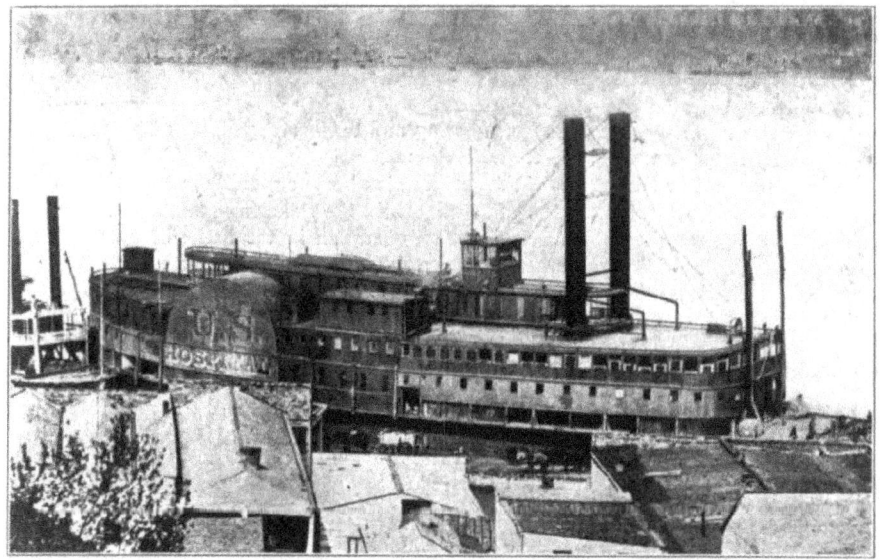

17-4: Hospital Transport Ship *Red Rover*

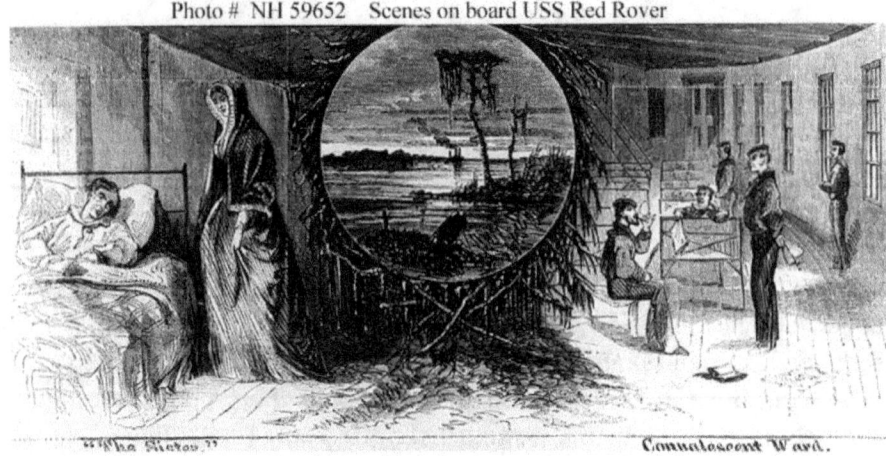

17-5: Hospital Transport Ship *Red Rover*

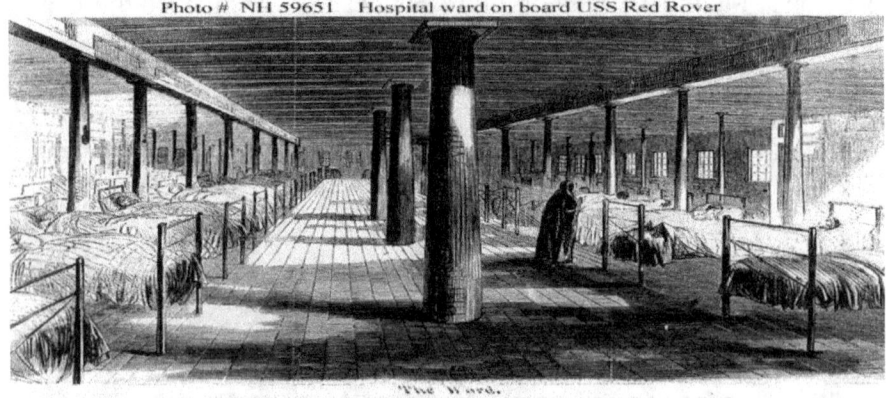

17-6: Hospital Transport Ship *Red Rover*

In an attempt to deal with the widespread instances of malaria among General Grant's troops in the Vicksburg Campaign, the steamer *Nashville* was called into action.

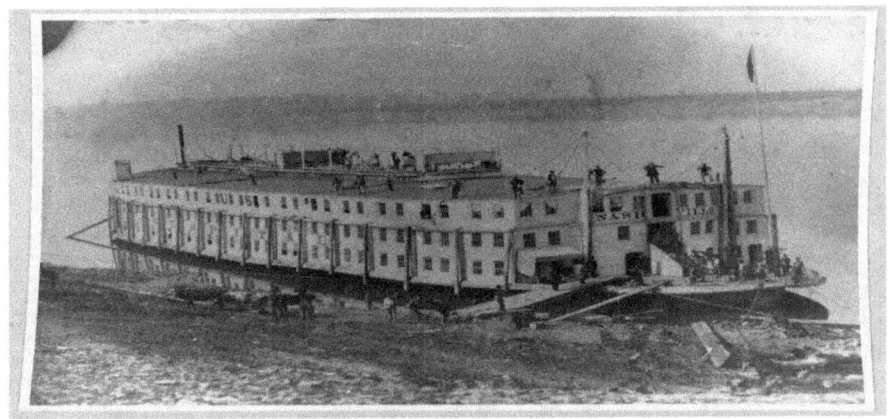

17-7: Hospital Transport Ship *Nashville*

Medical Director Charles MacDougall recognized the need for a floating hospital, in support of Grant's Vicksburg offensive, and arranged to have the hulk of the steamship *Nashville* outfitted as a 1,000-bed receiving hospital. The *Nashville* was eventually towed to Milliken's Bend, Louisiana where the swampy terrain had made medical care on shore impossible. The hospital vessel *D.A. January* was also moored at Milliken's Bend and acted as a floating hospital, as well. From March through June 1863, almost five thousand sick or wounded soldiers were admitted to the floating hospital; many were transferred to other vessels and carried to Memphis.

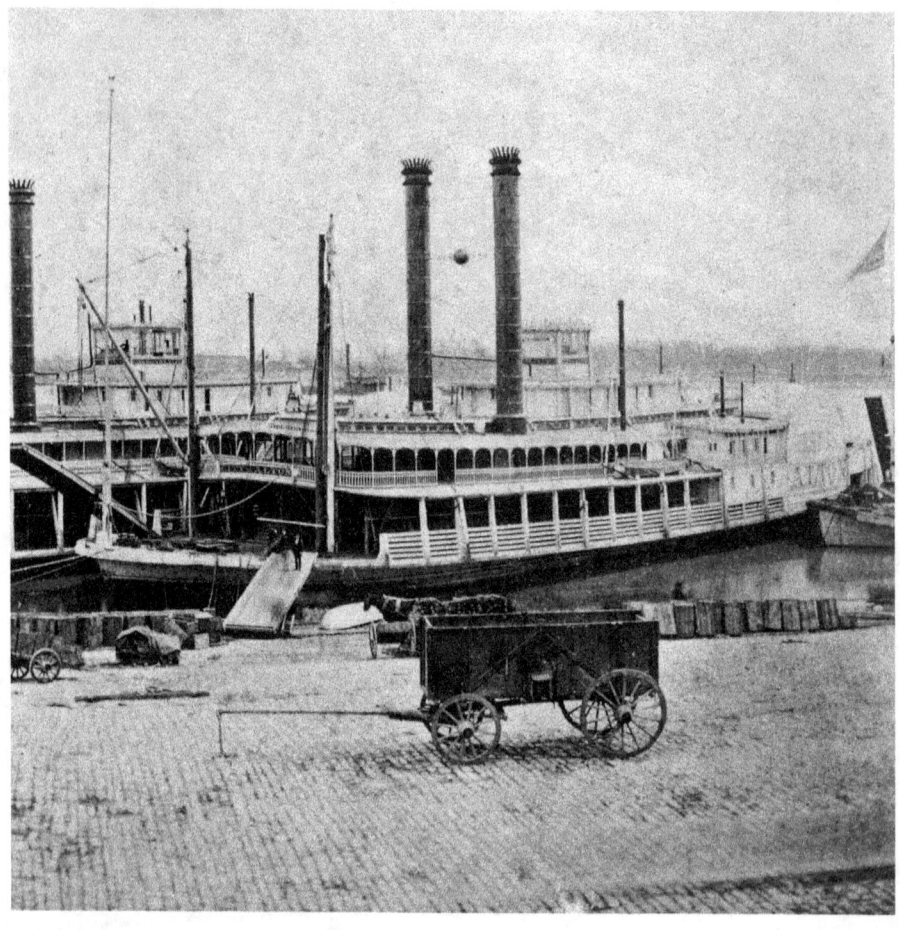

17-8: Hospital Transport Ship *City of Alton*

Here are bits of Emily Elizabeth Parsons's letters about serving as head nurse aboard the Hospital Steamship *City of Alton*:

> The ship was sent to Vicksburg, but its orders were changed at every stop, it seems. On their first trip they picked up hundreds of sick (as opposed to wounded) men at Helena and were instructed to take to Memphis, a hub of Union general hospitals. Then ship was ordered back to Vicksburg by General Grant where they witnessed preparation for fighting and saw from the river actual combat. She says to her parents that there is nothing like being in a War, it is indescribable and that the

wounds are like nothing she had seen in New England hospitals -- scrubbing floors and beds and doing laundry was a great part of Union hospital life, and it was a good thing because it introduced some small measure of sanitary conditions into the wards, even if the concept of "sterile" was a yet completely unknown.

In another letter, she explains that the hospital boats "steam under the yellow flag, and they do not usually fire upon that..."

She writes to her sister that "The hospital boats never take any part in the battle, or are fired upon as other boats are; the yellow flag floats at our mast-head to protect the wounded." Elsewhere she comments that there are no guns on the ship, however, if necessary, she believes she could find something.

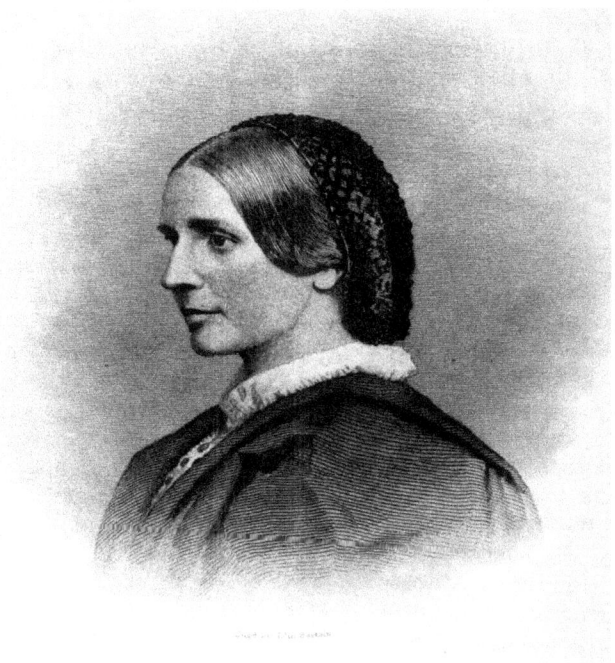

17-9: Emily E. Parsons

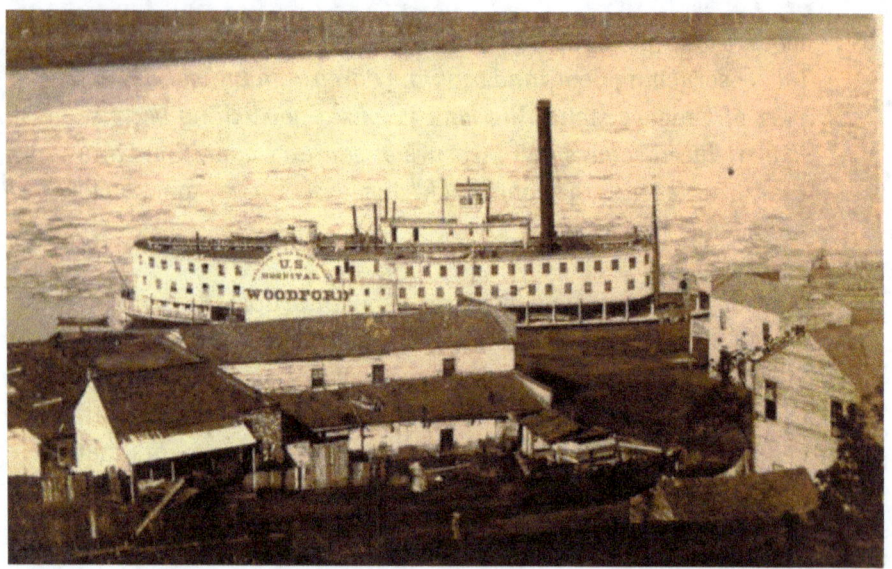

17-10: Hospital Transport Ship *Woodford* anchored on the Mississippi River at Vicksburg in January 1864.

CHAPTER 18
The Gettysburg Campaign

As the Harris railroad car was proving itself in the west, the largest evacuation of the wounded by rail up to that point occurred in the aftermath of the Battle of Gettysburg.

Of the 20,342 wounded that came under the care of the medical officers of the Army of the Potomac, 15,425 were evacuated by rail during the period from July 7-22, 1863 to general hospitals primarily located in Baltimore, York, Harrisburg, and New York City.

Let's take a look at the railroad infrastructure, in 1863, which was to play a vital role in the handling and transportation of the Union and Confederate soldiers following the Battle of Gettysburg.

These are the principal railroads which played a vital role during the Gettysburg campaign, leading up to the actual battle, especially during the period from June 15-June 30, 1863. The Baltimore and Ohio Railroad operated from Baltimore westward into the Shenandoah Valley and southwest to Washington, D.C. The Western Maryland Railroad extended its operations from Baltimore to Westminster and Union Bridge, Maryland in 1862. The Gettysburg and Hanover Railroad operated from Gettysburg eastward to Hanover, Pennsylvania. The Littlestown Railroad operated between Littlestown, Pennsylvania to Hanover. The Hanover Branch Railroad operated between Hanover and Hanover Junction. The Northern Central Railway operated north from Hanover Junction to York and Harrisburg and south from Hanover Junction to Baltimore.

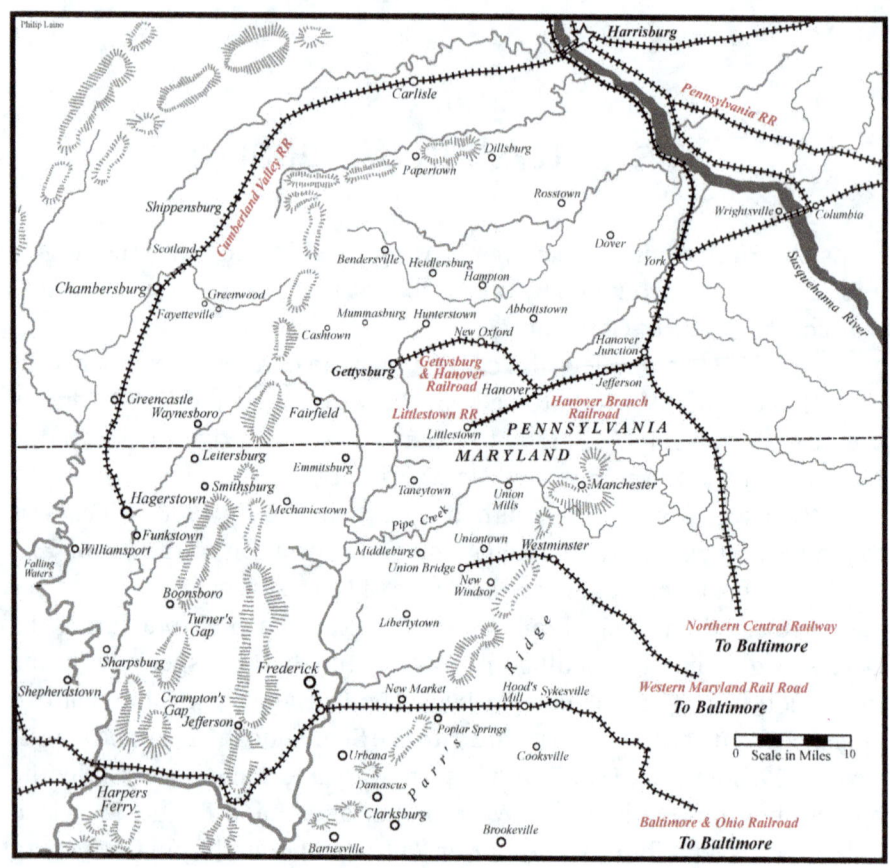

18-1: 1864 B & O Railroad Map

In downtown Baltimore, the Baltimore and Ohio Railroad operated out of the Camden Station located on Camden Street, the Northern Central Railway operated out of the Susquehanna Railroad Depot on Calvert Street, The Philadelphia and Baltimore Railroad operated out of the Philadelphia, Wilmington, and Baltimore Railroad Depot on the corner of President and Fleet Streets, and the Western Maryland Railway operated out of its Hillen Station located on Hillen Street. There was no rail connection between these four Baltimore stations, so passengers traveling north from Washington or south to Washington had to travel by horse-drawn wagons or carts or walk between stations in order to make connections. This, of course, made it very difficult for wounded soldiers to transfer from one railroad to another if they were traveling to general hospitals in various cities served by these different railroads.

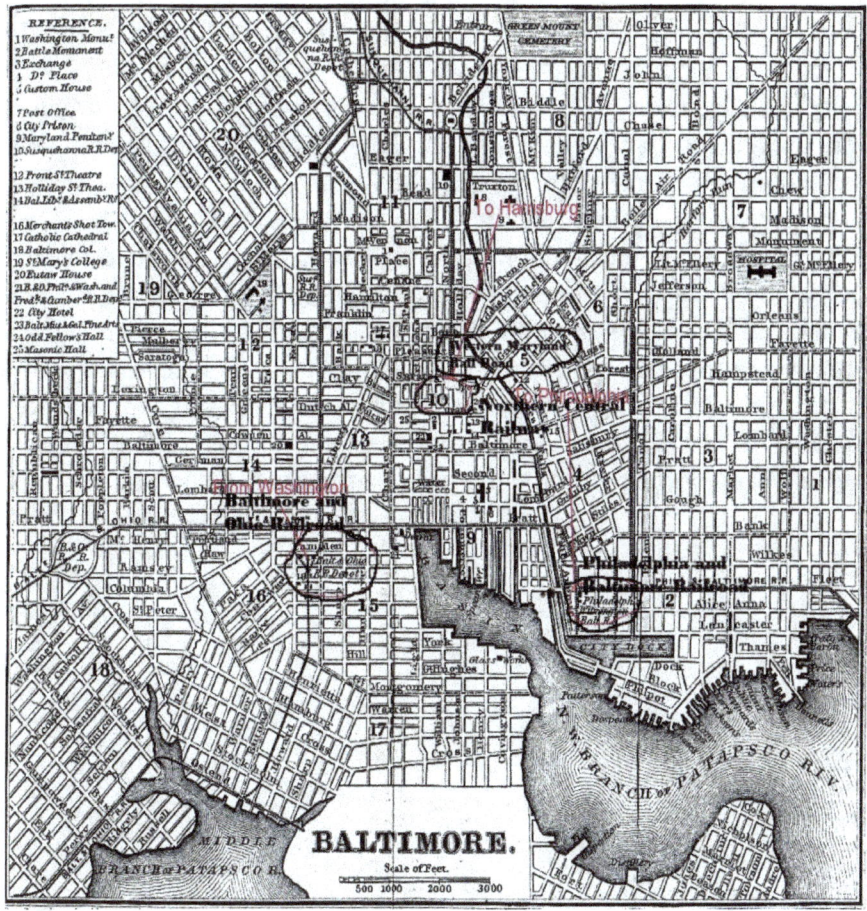

18-2: Baltimore, Maryland

After experiencing back-to-back victories at Fredericksburg and Chancellorsville, General Robert E. Lee looked to invade Pennsylvania. In the fulfillment of this quest, in Mid-June 1863, he ordered the destruction of B&O Railroad operations west of Martinsburg, West Virginia in order to defend his left flank as he would use the Blue Ridge Mountains to shield his right flank as he moved north through the Shenandoah Valley. With the destruction of B&O rails and other infrastructure, Lee focused on doing the same to rail operations in the north. Once he entered Pennsylvania, on June 23, Confederate Major General Jubal Early's 35th Battalion of Virginia Cavalry and the 17th Virginia Cavalry were dispatched to destroy various strategic railroad bridges and other infrastructure belonging to the Gettysburg and Hanover Railroad, Hanover Branch Railroad and the Northern Central Railway. On June 27, 1863, Early's cavalry burned the covered bridge over Rock Creek, east of Gettysburg, and the New Oxford Bridge over the Canewago Creek. Both railroad bridges are along the Gettysburg and Hanover Railroad. This vital artery would remain closed for days after the battle while the U.S. Military Railroad, under the direction of its Chief Engineer Union General Herman Haupt hastened to make the necessary repairs to these torched bridges. Continuing east, on June 28 and 29, Early's cavalry raided the facilities of the Northern Central Railway and the Hanover Branch Railroad. In his brief occupation of York (June 28-30, 1863), his troops burned a dozen bridges as far as York Haven and all nineteen bridges on the Wrightville spur. The loss of these bridges effectively impaired rail traffic between Baltimore and Harrisburg.

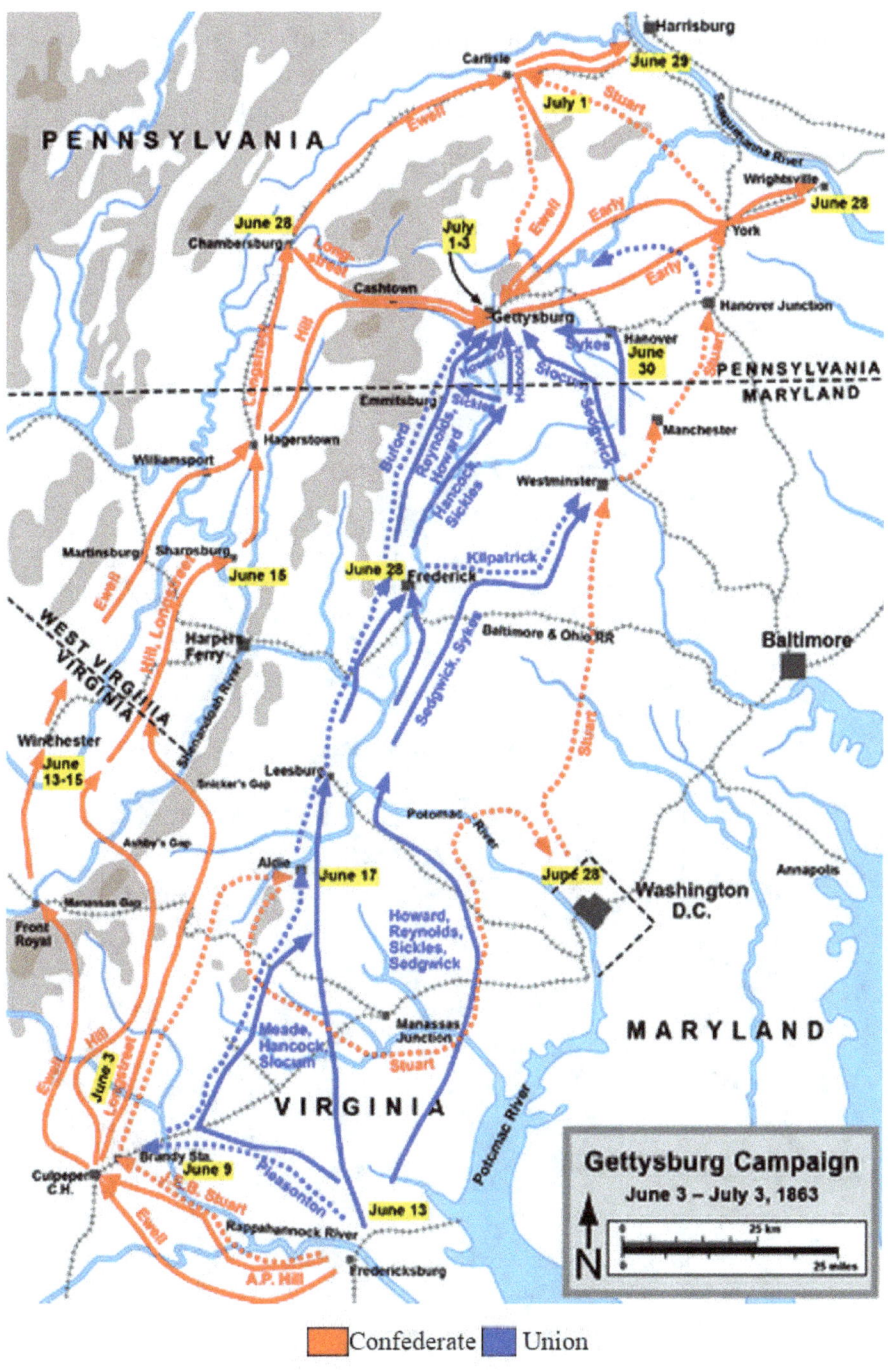

18-3: The Gettysburg Campaign

126 | Hospital Trains and Vessels during the Civil War

The following map was made for the benefit of General George Meade, the newly appointed Commander of the Army of the Potomac, showing the damage to rail bridges attributed to the raids of General Early's Cavalry during the Gettysburg Campaign.

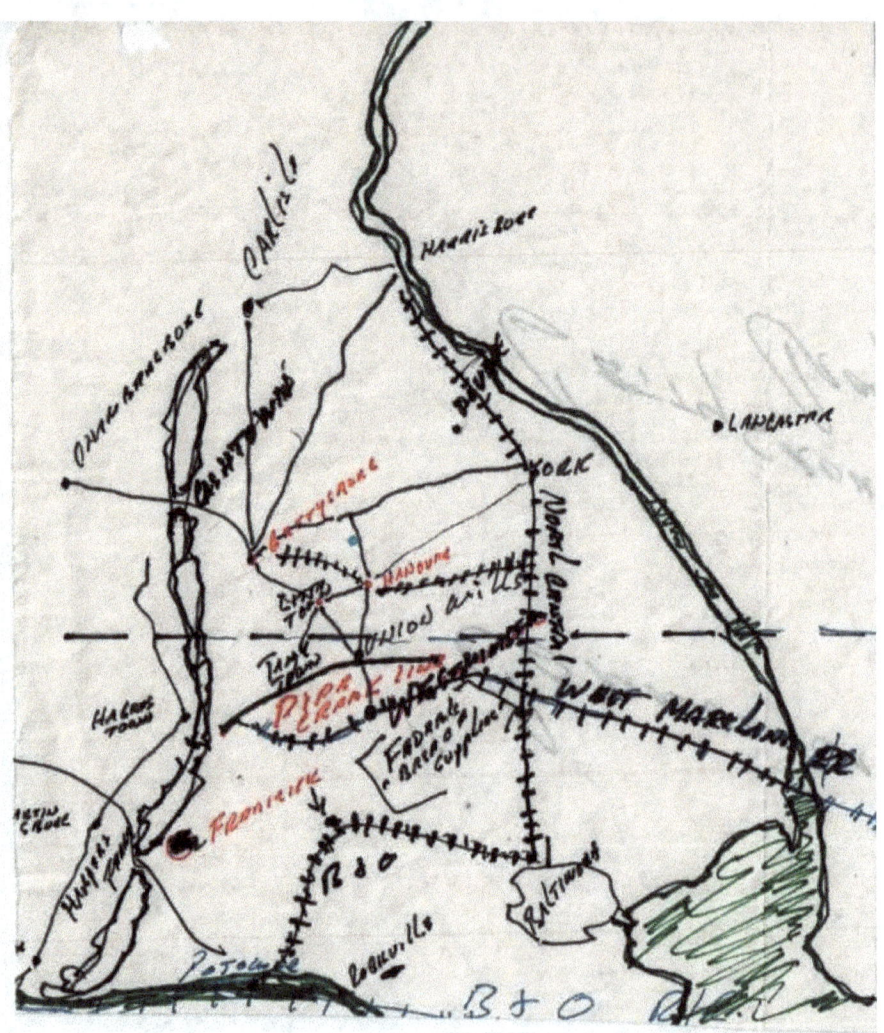

18-4: Gen. Meade's map showing damage to rail bridges during the Gettysburg Campaign

The following is a Report of Maj. Gen. Jubal A. Early, C. S. Army, commanding division.

JUNE 3–AUGUST 1, 1863.
The Gettysburg Campaign. O.R.
SERIES I, VOLUME XXVII/2 [S# 44]
HEADQUARTERS EARLY'S DIVISION

August 22, 1863.
Maj. A. S. PENDLETON,
Asst. Adjt. Gen., Second Corps. Army of Northern Virginia.

The authorities of Gettysburg declared their inability to furnish any supplies, and a search of the stores resulted in securing only a very small quantity of commissary supplies, and about 2,000 rations were found in a train of cars, and issued to Gordon's brigade. The cars, numbering 10 or 12, were burned, as was also a small railroad bridge (Rock Creek) near the place. I ordered Tanner's battery of Jones' battalion, to report to General Gordon during the night, and also a company of French's cavalry, and directed him to move with them and his brigade on the turnpike toward York at light next morning, and I also directed Colonel White to proceed with his cavalry to Hanover Junction, on the Northern Central road, destroying the railroad bridges on the way, and to destroy the junction and a bridge or two south of it, and then proceed toward York, burning all the bridges up to that place.

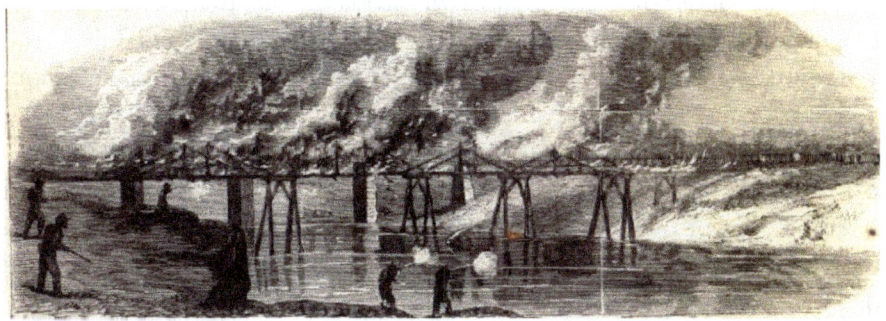

18-5: Railway bridge burning

In his brief occupation of York (June 28-30, 1863), Early's troops burned a dozen bridges on the Northern Central Railway as far as York Haven and all nineteen bridges on the Wrightville spur. The Northern Central Railway ran a spur from York to Wrightsville which connected with the Pennsylvania Railroad using the Columbia Bridge. The loss of these bridges effectively impaired all rail traffic between Baltimore and Harrisburg.

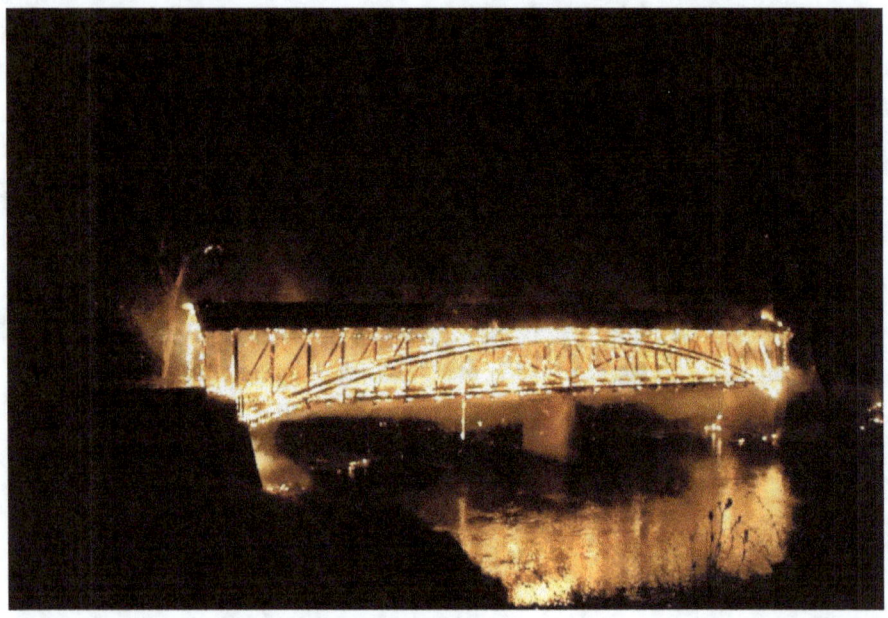

18-6: Railway bridge burning

The alternate rail route had its own problems due to operational deficiencies rather than to physical damage by the enemy. On July 1, the very same day the epic battle at Gettysburg began, Haupt made a personal inspection of the Western Maryland Railroad line. By the time he arrived in Westminster, it was crystal clear that he was facing the greatest challenge of his military career. The Western Maryland Railroad had been taken over by Federal authorities, under the auspices of the United States Military Railroad on June 28, 1863, because of its strategic location as the main supply route for the entire Union army, under General George Meade, that was amassing in the Westminster/Carroll County area prior to the battle. Westminster was the closest rail terminal to Gettysburg. From there, it was twenty miles of road to the site of the battlefield. There were reported to be 5,000 army wagons, with 12,000 troops operating in the Westminster area at the time. Despite this criticality to the Union cause, what General Haupt found was a single-track, 29-mile-long railroad in relatively poor condition operating between Relay House, on the Northern Central Railway line, and Westminster. There were no sidings for long trains, turntables, water stations or telegraph. At best, the Western Maryland could handle four trains a day which was totally inadequate to supply the army. In order to rectify this situation, he immediately brought in his Construction Corps in order to bring the railroad up to speed. Sufficient locomotives, cars, fuel, supplies to operate it were brought in to support their efforts.

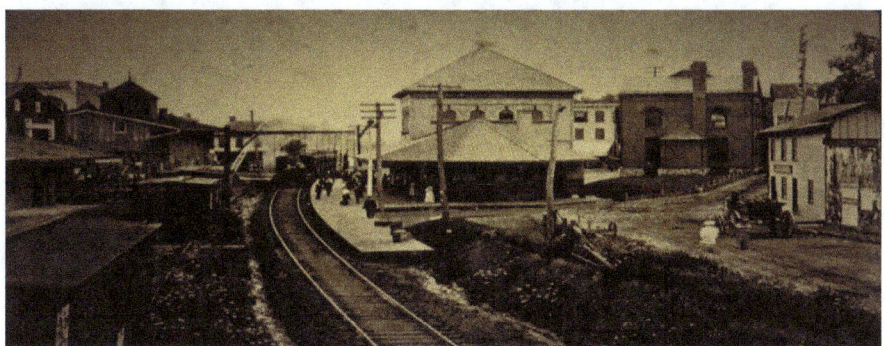

18-7: Westminster Station

Figure 18-8 shows General Haupt himself, standing on the small hill to the right, supervising embankment work and rail repair. The locomotive "General Haupt" was named after its namesake and was used by him as he supervised various rail operations which included, among other things the emergency refurbishing of the Western Maryland Railroad.

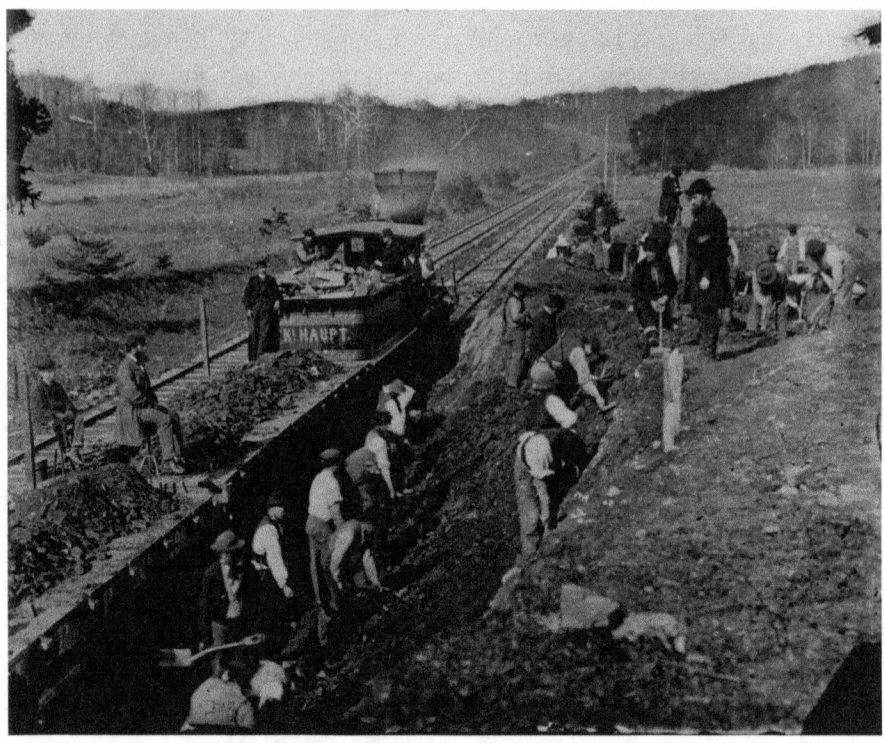

18-8: Gen. Haupt supervising rail repair

The Battle of Gettysburg was fought from July 1–3, 1863 in and around the town of Gettysburg, Pennsylvania involving 104,256 Union forces and from 71,000-75,000 Confederate forces. The battle involved the largest number of casualties of the entire war and is often described as the war's turning point. Union Major General George Meade's Army of the Potomac defeated attacks by Confederate Gen. Robert E. Lee's Army of Northern Virginia, halting Lee's invasion of the North. During the three day battle at Gettysburg, July 1-3, 1863, it is estimated that 33,264 soldiers were wounded (14,529 Union and 18,735 Confederate). On July 3, 1863 after the collapse of Pickett, Pettigrew and Trimble's valiant charge, the Gettysburg area was one vast field hospital with wounded Union and Confederate soldiers lying in every structure, in the fields, in the woods, and directly in the summer. The treatment of the wounded at Gettysburg after the battle was left up to the mercy of the Army of the Potomac, as well as the good citizens of Gettysburg, and the flock of both local and out-of-town nurses who voluntarily came to Gettysburg to help the stricken soldiers on both sides of the battlefield. The US Sanitary Commission, a voluntary relief organization, played a vital role on the battlefield, at field hospitals and along the train route where the wounded where transported. Also important to note are the communities of religious women – such as the Daughters of Charity – who took part in the care of wounded and sick on battlefields, in hospitals, camps, and prisons for both the Union and the Confederacy. As far as the military handling of these wounded, both Union and Confederate soldiers would have been treated and moved together. Once a soldier was wounded he was no longer considered the enemy. *The railroads which provided service in support of the Gettysburg Campaign with men, food and munitions were now called into service in order to evacuate the multitude of wounded.*

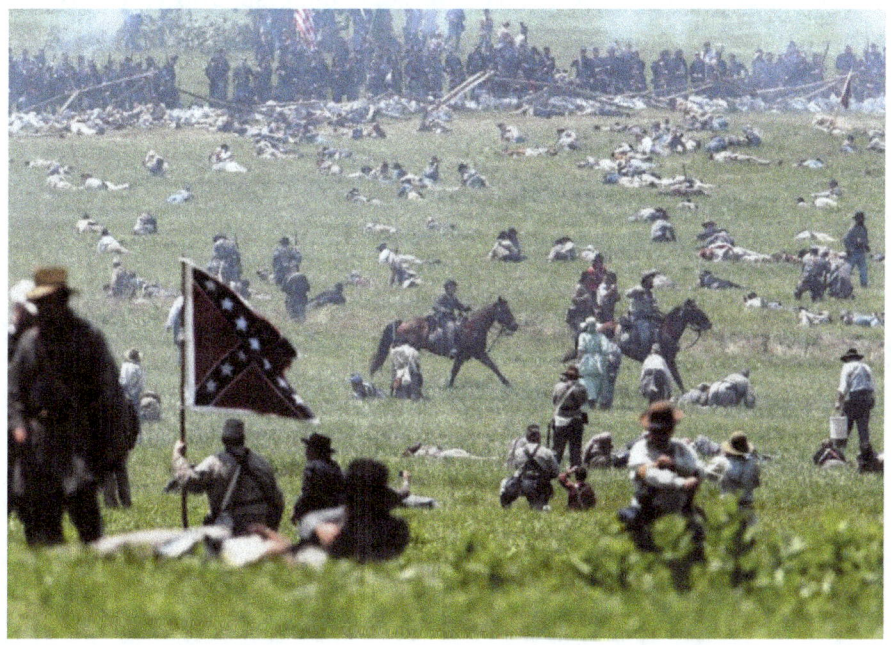

18-9: "Wounded" Civil War re-enactors litter the Gettysburg battlefield at the end of Pickett's Charge on June 30, 2013

Thanks to the valiant efforts of the Ambulance Corps, the field of battle was quickly cleared of the wounded. According to the *Report on Medical Operations at Gettysburg* written by Dr. Jonathan A. Letterman:

> "The ambulance corps throughout the army acted in the most commendable manner during those days of severe labor. Notwithstanding the great number of wounded... I have it from the most reliable authority and from my own observation that not one wounded man of all that number was left on the field within our (Union) lines early on the morning of July 4."

Following the battle, and after assessing the logistical challenges offered by the Western Maryland Railroad, General Haupt, from his vantage point in Westminster, was able to operate a total of 30 trains a day (15 each way), running in convoys of up to five trains at a time between Baltimore and Westminster on eight hour shifts on the Western Maryland Railroad. In order to insure that the convoys ran on schedule, Haupt ordered his chief conduction engineer, Adria Anderson, to bring a train to Baltimore with 400 men equipped with an ample supply of buckets, lanterns and pre-cut firewood for the locomotives. Crews would be dropped off between the Relay House on the Northern Central Railway and Westminster with piles of wood to resupply the tenders. Lacking any water stations in Westminster, other crews would be positioned near streams to provide bucket brigades to refill the water tanks on the engines. The lanterns would allow for twenty-four operation if required. The trains brought in fifteen hundred tons of supplies per day and returned with thousands of wounded soldiers. Since there was no turntable at Westminster, trains made the return trip in reverse.

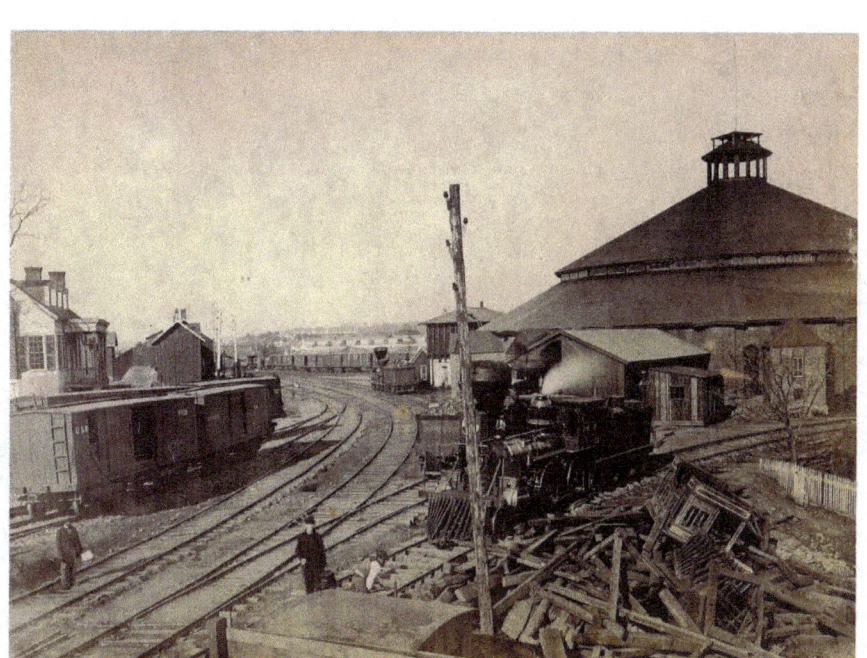

18-10: Roundhouse

Following the battle, the Western Maryland Railroad was returned to the civilian owners on July 7, 1863 after most of the injured were transported. Both the Western Maryland Railroad stations at Westminster and Union Bridge were used after the Battle of Gettysburg to move wounded soldiers from ambulance wagons and load them onto trains destined for hospitals in Baltimore.

According to the *Report on the Transportation of Wounded after the Battle of Gettysburg*, prepared by E.P. Vollum, the U.S. Army Medical Officer, about 2,000 wounded Union soldiers were transported from Westminster to Baltimore. To this day, one (sometimes erroneously identified as more than one) of the railroad tracks southeast of the former Western Maryland Union Bridge station is still identified as the "Hospital Track."

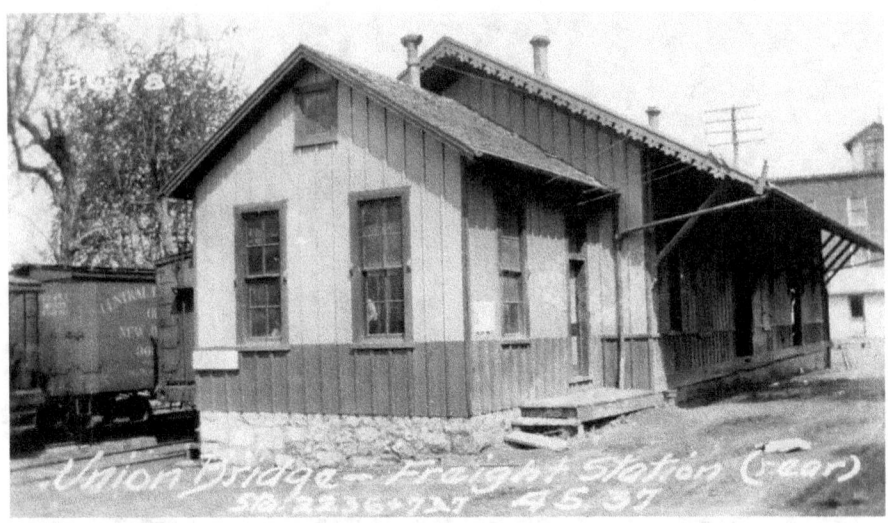

18-11: Union Bridge Station

On their return trip from Baltimore, trains carried fresh troops, gun powder, food and bandages back to Westminster.

The use of the Western Maryland Railroad, in the evacuation of the wounded from Gettysburg, was often more expeditious than the Gettysburg and Hanover Railroad, Hanover Branch Railroad and Northern Central Railroad route which often experience "bottlenecks" and delays.

Due to the large number of wounded soldiers, resulting from the Battle of Gettysburg, private residences and farms were all converted to field hospitals once the sheer magnitude of number of wounded was realized. According to Union Major Dr. Jonathan Letterman, the Medical Director for the Army of the Potomac, 6 ambulance and 4 wagons from each Corps were left behind, after the battle, to take the wounded from the field hospitals to the Gettysburg railroad depot or, as more commonly known as, the Gettysburg Railroad Station. Although it is commonly believed that the station was used as a field hospital following the battle, this was not its original purpose. It was intended to be only a transit place, although it is likely that some re-bandaging of wounds and other care was administered before the wounded soldiers were transported. This sketch of the barricade at the Railroad Depot in Gettysburg (to the right) was made circa July 1-3, 1863. The barricade was constructed of timber, old carts and so forth. The sketch was made by Alfred R. Waud who was famous for his Civil War sketches.

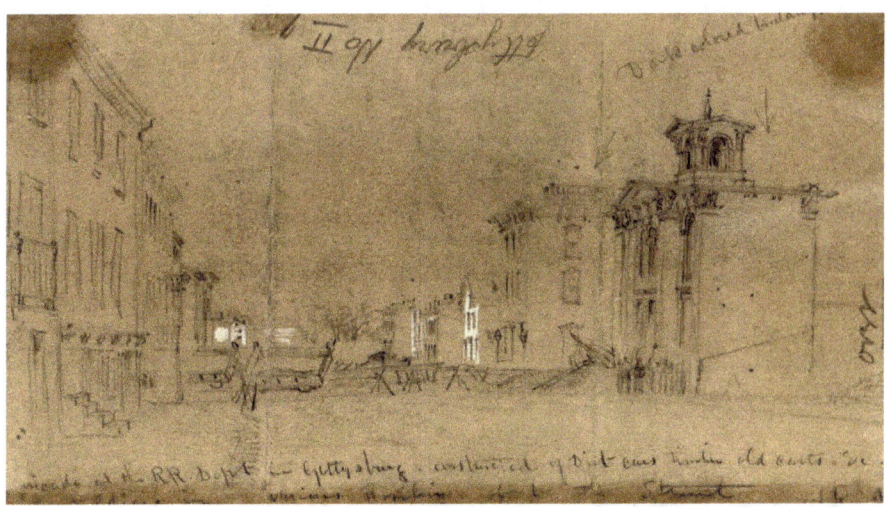

18-12: Barricade at the railroad depot in
Gettysburg, Alfred R. Waud.

On July 7, 1863, just three days after the fighting ended at Gettysburg, Haupt's construction crews had brought the railroad tracks to the outskirts of Gettysburg. The bridge over Rock Creek which ran east of town still needed repair (the Confederates had burned it on June 26th, but Haupt, confident the military quartermasters in Gettysburg could oversee that final project, headed back to Washington to report on the situation. On July 9, 1863, despite General Haupt's assertions to the contrary, his crews still hadn't repaired the Rock Creek Bridge, burned on June 27 along with seventeen railroad cars, with needed supplies pushed off the trains into the nearby fields and 4,000 wounded men waiting for transportation at the Gettysburg Railroad Station.

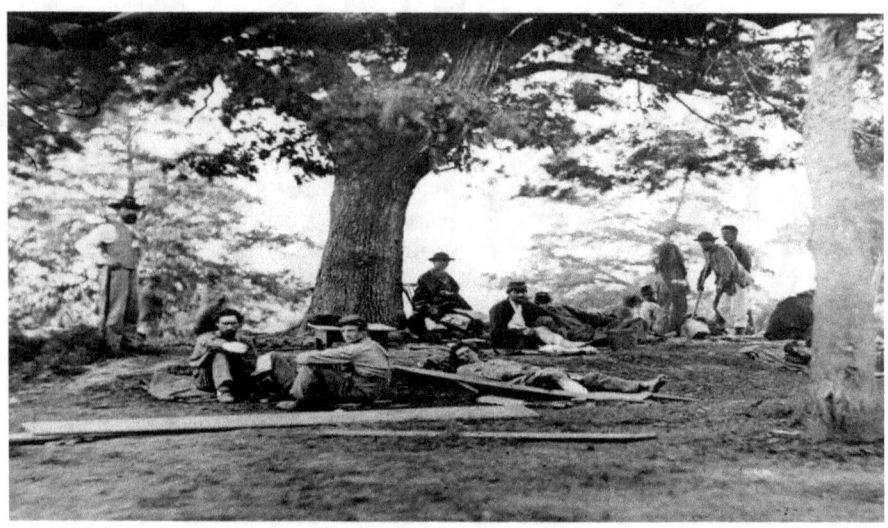

18-13: Wounded waiting for transport from Gettysburg

Until the bridge was repaired, the only wounded soldiers that could be moved from the Gettysburg area, from July 7 until July 9, were from Camp Letterman which was located east of the destroyed Rock Creek Bridge. It was a full week since the battle before regular train service was restored to Gettysburg.

Sanitary Commission nurse Georgeanna Woolsey described it in this way in her recollections entitled *Three Weeks at Gettysburg*: "The railroad bridge broken up the enemy, Government had not rebuilt a yet, and we stopped two miles from town, to find that, as usual, just where the Government had left off the Commission had come in. There stood their temporary lodge at kitchen and here hobbling out of their tents came the wounded who had made their way down from the Corps hospital (Camp Letterman) expecting to leave once in return cars. This is the way the thing was managed at first: the surgeons left in care of the wounded three or four miles out from the town, went up and down among the men in the morning, and said: Any of you boys who can make your way to the cars (railroad), can go to Baltimore."

In an attempt to elevate the suffering of the wounded flowing into the Gettysburg Railroad Station and its environs, the U.S. Sanitary Commission erected large tents in order to receive and refresh the wounded while they waited to be evacuated by rail.

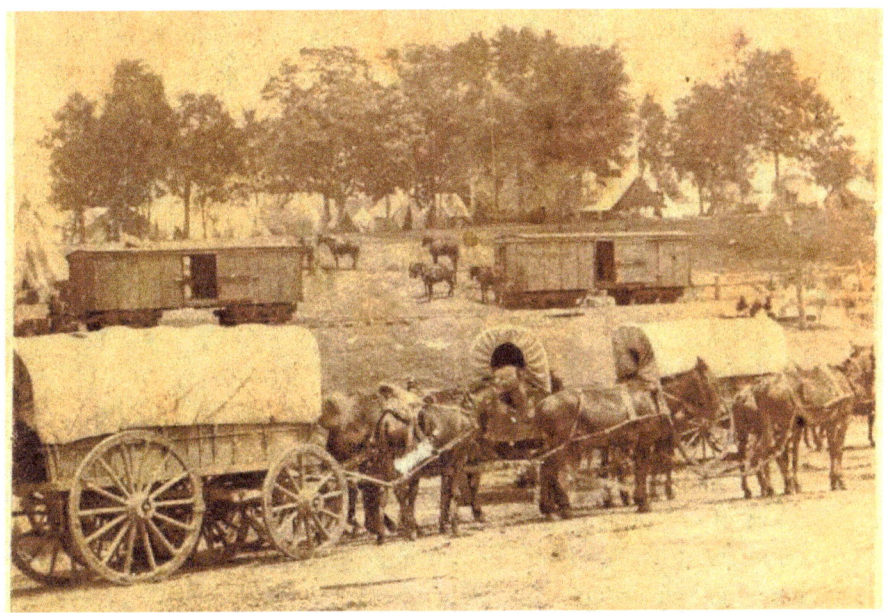

18-14: Savage Station

Livid with this situation at the railroad station, Haupt seized full military possession of the 30 mile rail line, from the civilian operators, from Hanover Junction to Gettysburg until August 4. Determined to make things right, Haupt would personally oversee the repairs of the bridge and the reopening of the rail line from the Gettysburg depot on July 10. His primary goal was to remove wounded soldiers from the field of battle, through the depot, to distant hospitals. During the military occupation, 11,425 wounded men were so transported. The station was always crowded with wounded waiting for trains that departed at least twice a day, carrying their passengers towards home or to distant hospitals. Inbound trains delivered medical supplies and brought volunteers to help the wounded. Haupt would personally oversee the repairs to the Rock Creek Bridge. However, the initial repairs to this and other bridges were only temporary in order to expedite the evacuation of wounded soldiers from Gettysburg. Therefore, initially only lighter weight locomotives, traveling at reduced speeds, could be used when crossing these bridges. Before the Rock Creek Bridge was repaired, he set up a schedule whereby trains left the Camp Letterman depot twice a day at 10 AM and 5 PM.

Once this bridge was reopened, General Haupt took personal charge of setting up a schedule for the timely evacuation of the wounded out of the Gettysburg station itself. Beginning on July 10, trains carried the injured from Gettysburg's depot on N. Carlisle Street, at least twice a day, in the morning and afternoon, stopping at Camp Letterman before continuing its journey eastward. Additional trains would be added and the schedule adjusted as needed over the next three weeks.

In Vollum's *Report*, he states:

> "...every train of wounded was placed in (the) charge of a medical officer.... Instruments, dressings, Stimulants, etc., were furnished him, and he was instructed to announce his coming by telegraph, if possible, and report to the Medical Director at the place of his destination. Each car was filled with a sufficient quantity of hay, and, on longer routes, water coolers, tin cups, bedpans and urinals were placed in them, and guarded on the route by some agents of the Sanitary Commission. In some instances, these conveniences were furnished by the medical department, but the demand for them by the hospitals often exhausted the supplies of the purveyors. Before leaving, the wounded were fed and watered by the Sanitary Commission, and often hundreds of wounded, laid over for a night or part of the day, were attended and fed by the commission whose agents placed them in the cars."

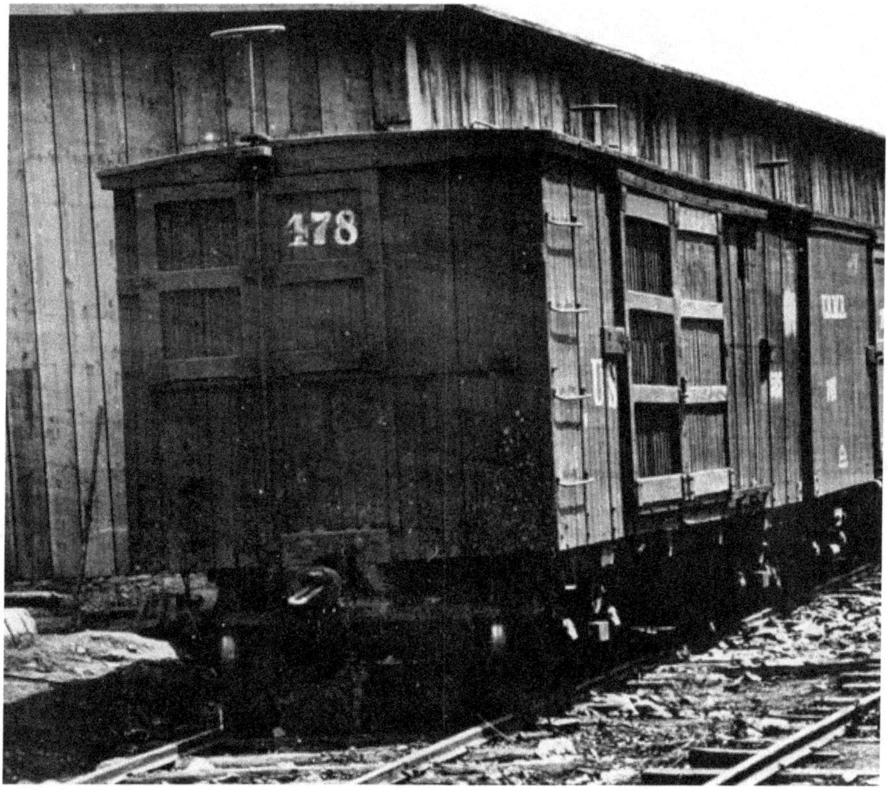

18-15: Vented box cars

According to the Vollum's *Report*, the following tabulation shows the number and destination of Union and Confederate wounded sent from Gettysburg from July 7-22, 1863. All told, more than 11,000 wounded men left the Gettysburg area via Hanover Junction between July 7 and July 22 mostly traveling to Baltimore.

DATE	TRAIN	NO.	DESCRIPTION	DESTINATION	TOTAL PER DIEM	DATE	TRAIN	NO.	DESCRIPTION	DESTINATION	TOTAL PER DIEM
1863.						1863.					
July 7	5 P.M.	164	Union	Baltimore		July 15	.. .. ..	6	Confederate	Baltimore	603
" 7	7 P.M.	258	"	"		" 16	9 A.M.	60	Union	"	
" 7	7.10 P.M.	400	"	"	822	" 16	3 P.M.	36	"	"	
" 8	1.40 P.M.	640	"	"	640	" 16	.. .. ..	262	Confederate	"	358
" 9	10.35 A.M.	3,012	"	"		" 17	9 A.M.	20	Union	New York	
" 9	5.30 P.M.	1,061	"	"	2,073	" 17	.. .. ..	225	Confederate	"	
" 10	11 A.M.	186	"	"		" 17	.. .. ..	204	"	"	
" 10	5.15 P.M.	620	"	"	806	" 17	.. .. ..	80	Union	York, Penn.	529
" 11	11 A.M.	204	"	"		" 18	9 A.M.	47	"	"	
" 11	5 P.M.	338	"	"		" 18	.. .. ..	183	Confederate	Baltimore	
" 11	5 P.M.	76	Confederate	"	618	" 18	3 P.M.	125	Union	York, Penn.	
" 12	10 A.M.	327	"	"		" 18	.. .. ..	350	Confederate	Baltimore	705
" 12	.. .. ..	28	Union	"		" 19	9 A.M.	107	Union	York, Penn.	
" 12	12.15 P.M.	142	"	"		" 19	.. .. ..	25	Confederate	"	
" 12	.. .. ..	184	Confederate	"		" 19	3 P.M.	198	Union	"	
" 12	5 P.M.	105	Union	"		" 19	.. .. ..	125	Confederate	Baltimore	455
" 12	.. .. ..	433	Confederate	"	1,219	" 20	9 A.M.	257	Union	York, Penn.	
" 13	9 A.M.	06	Union	"		" 20	3 P.M.	141	"	"	398
" 13	.. .. ..	133	Confederate	"		" 21	11.30 A.M.	467	Confederate	New York	
" 13	3 P.M.	259	Union	"		" 21	.. .. ..	33	Union	"	
" 13	.. .. ..	16	Confederate	"	504	" 21	4 P.M.	158	Confederate	"	
" 14	9 A.M.	180	Union	"		" 21	.. .. ..	54	Union	York, Penn.	712
" 14	3 P.M.	176	"	"		" 22	11.30 A.M.	47	"	Harrisburg	
" 14	.. .. ..	394	Confederate	"	700	" 22	.. .. ..	154	Confederate	New York	
" 15	9 A.M.	182	Union	"		" 22	4 P.M.	22	Union	Harrisburg	
" 15	.. .. ..	37	Confederate	"		" 22	.. .. ..	58	Confederate	New York	281
" 15	3 P.M.	380	Union	"				11,425			11,425

Wounded sent from Gettysburg to 22d instant:

Union 7,608
Confederate 3,817
Total 11,425

18-16: *Wounded sent from Gettysburg, July 7-22, 1863*

On July 9, over two thousand soldiers were sent to Baltimore and on July 12, the next busiest day, 1,219 soldiers were sent to Baltimore on three different trains. On the other days, the daily number of soldiers shipped to the rear ranged from 300 to 800. The journey required the collaboration of the medical department, the quartermaster's corps and various civilian relief agencies.

As mentioned earlier, the other location where wounded Union and Confederate soldiers were evaluated by rail was at Camp Letterman located northeast of the Gettysburg battlefield and established on July 5, 1863.

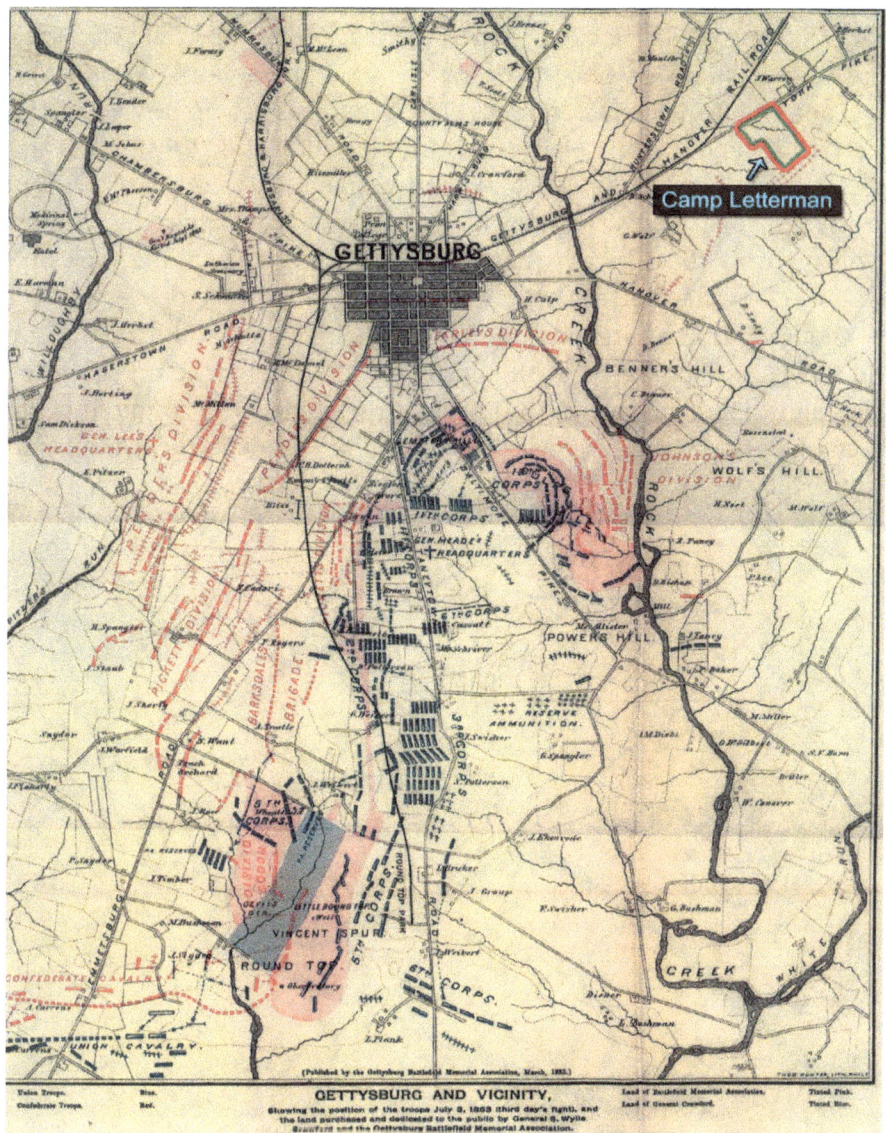

18-17: Camp Letterman

Camp Lettermen, named after Medical Director for the Army of the Potomac, served the large number of wounded that were recuperating from surgery and provided "the bridge in medical treatment" between the field hospitals around Gettysburg and the large, permanent general or base hospitals located in metropolitan areas. The camp is often referred to as a "Train Ready" hospital where patients were medically stabilized for their train ride to general hospitals in Baltimore, York, Washington, D.C and other metropolitan areas. The camp was set up in view of the Gettysburg and Hanover Railroad which brought in medical supplies and took out wounded men following their treatment at the Camp.

Georgeanna Woolsey came to Gettysburg accompanied by another woman from the Sanitary Commission, to assist with the sick and wounded at Camp Letterman.

Along with the surgeons located there, their main duty during the three weeks they stayed at the hospital was to help feed and care for the multitude of Union and Confederate wounded who came into the "Sanitary Lodge" located near temporary railroad depot near the camp where they were fed and treated.

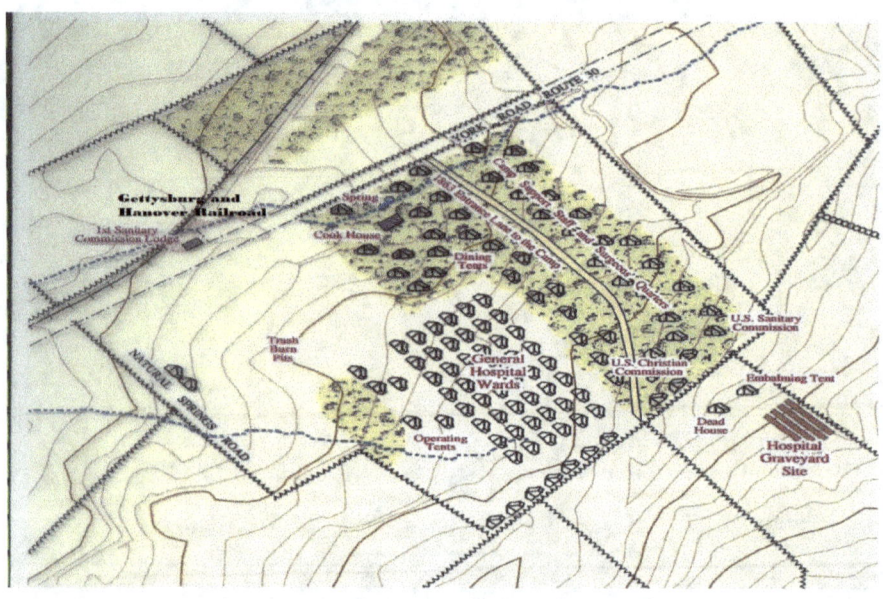

18-18: Camp Letterman

Here the wounded men waited for the next train to take them out of the Camp to hospitals in Baltimore and Philadelphia. Since the trains originated from the Gettysburg depot, the trains arriving at Camp Letterman were sometimes already full and the wounded soldiers had to spend the night by the rail line. She estimated that in the three weeks after the Camp was established; she served sixteen thousand meals and arranged for a night's sleep for four thousand wounded soldiers who were evacuated from the Camp.

> "Things were systemized now," [Woolsey wrote], "...and the men came down in long ambulance trains to the cars; baggage-cars they were, filled with straw for the wounded to lie in, and broken open at either end to let in the air... When the surgeons had all the wounded placed, with as much comfort as seemed possible under the circumstances, on board the train, our detail of men would go from car to car, with soup made of beef-stock or fresh meat, full of potatoes, turnips, cabbage and rice, with fresh bread and coffee, and, when stimulants were needed, with ale, milk-punch, or brandy."

This facility would treat more than 14,000 Union and 6,800 Confederate wounded as a result of the battle. The camp remained at Gettysburg until November 1863 when the last remaining patients left, the tents were packed, and the doctors and nurses left for other battlefield hospitals.

Haupt and his construction crew eventually completely rebuilt all 19 bridges belong to the Northern Central Railway with the help of the railway itself. Additional bridges along the Wrightsville spur would be rebuilt by August with the help of the Northern Central Railway.

The following Mathew Brady photograph shows the rebuilt Northern Central Railway Bridge over the Codorus Creek at Hanover Junction. Confederate cavalrymen had destroyed the previous bridge during their June 1863 raid. By July 22, 1863, the Gettysburg and Hanover Railroad, the Hanover Branch Railroad and the Northern Central Railway were once again fully operational with completely new bridges replacing any temporary structures.

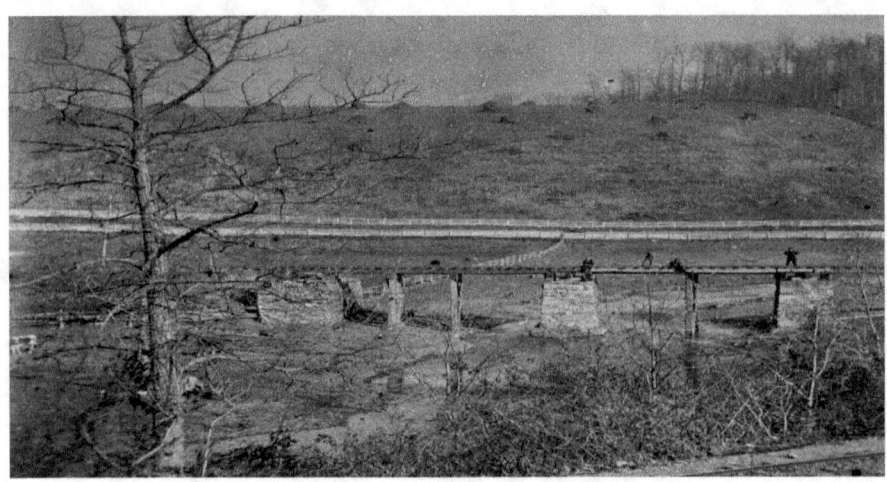

18-19: Northern Central Railway Bridge over the Codorus Creek at Hanover Junction.

The opening of the Northern Central Railway on July 22, 1863 meant that all rail traffic north to York and Harrisburg and south to Baltimore was now fully operational.

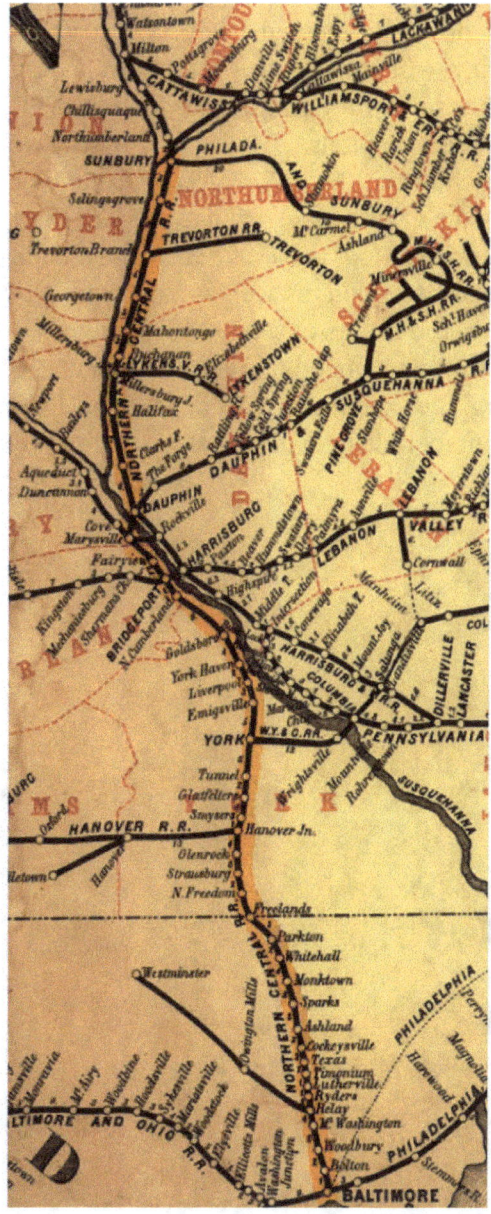

18-20: Northern Central Railway line

Those wounded soldiers transported from Gettysburg via the Gettysburg and Hanover and Hanover Branch Railroads all disembarked at Hanover Junction. There, the Northern Central Railway would them to large general hospitals located in York, Harrisburg and Baltimore. In Baltimore, they would take the Baltimore and Ohio Railroad to Washington, D.C. hospitals or take the Philadelphia and Baltimore Railroad to Philadelphia-based hospitals.

At the Hanover Junction, the U.S. Christian Commission set up aid stations in box cars on a rail siding. Trains stopping there contained from 300 to 800 of the wounded, some of which were badly wounded. They were given medical attention, as well as beverages, soft bread and biscuits. At Baltimore, the agents of several benevolent societies distributed food bountifully to the wounded in the cars immediately on their arrival; and at Harrisburg, the commissary department had made arrangements for feeding any number likely to pass that way.

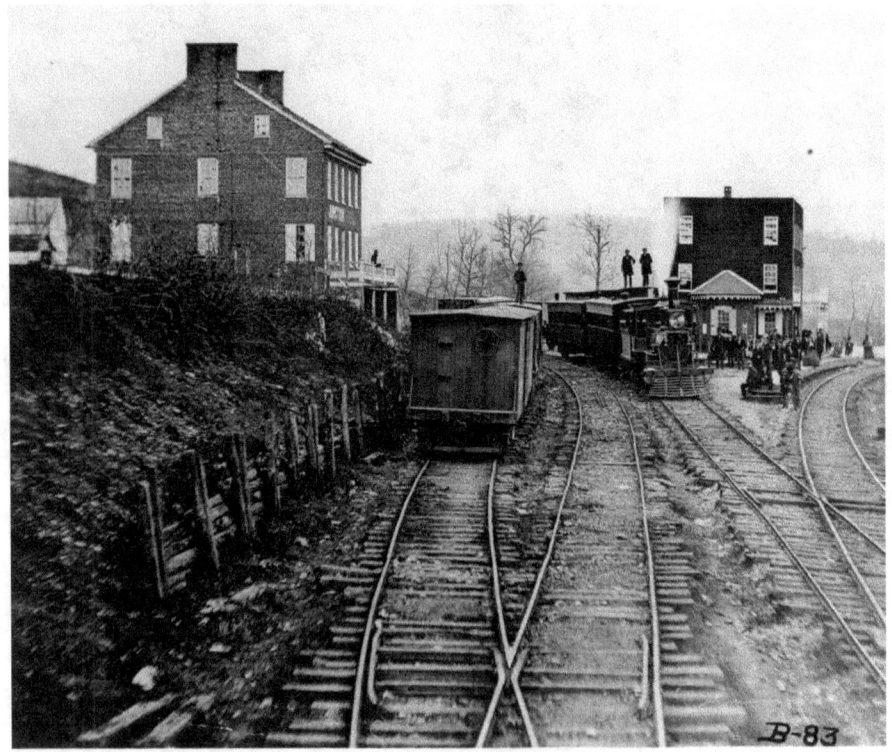

18-21: Hanover Junction

No discussion about the care of wounded soldiers, following the Battle of Gettysburg, would be complete without a discussion of the important role of the town of Littlestown, Pennsylvania. Littlestown is located ten miles southeast of Gettysburg and seven miles southwest of Hanover. It played a vital part in the Civil War, especially during and following the Battle of Gettysburg. A band of Confederates entered Littlestown on the morning of June 26, 1863, the advance of Early's Division, Ewell's Corps, the Army of the Northern Virginia, which was crossing the Maryland line into Pennsylvania.

After the battle, hundreds of wounded soldiers were brought in ambulances from Gettysburg and placed on the railroad cars at Littlestown. General Daniel E. Sickles, who had lost a leg at Round Top during the Battle of Gettysburg, was among the wounded treated in Littlestown at a local hospital before being transported to Hanover. The Littlestown Branch Railroad, or simply the Littlestown Railroad, would be a major player in this event. The railroad founded on July 1, 1858, was a subsidiary of the Pennsylvania Railroad, for the seven mile stretch from Littlestown to Hanover. The Pennsylvania Railroad Station at Littlestown is now shown. It was observed in Vollum's *Report*, that approximately 2,000 wounded Union soldiers were transported from Littlestown to large general hospitals in Baltimore via the Littlestown Railroad, Hanover Branch Railroad and the Northern Central Railway.

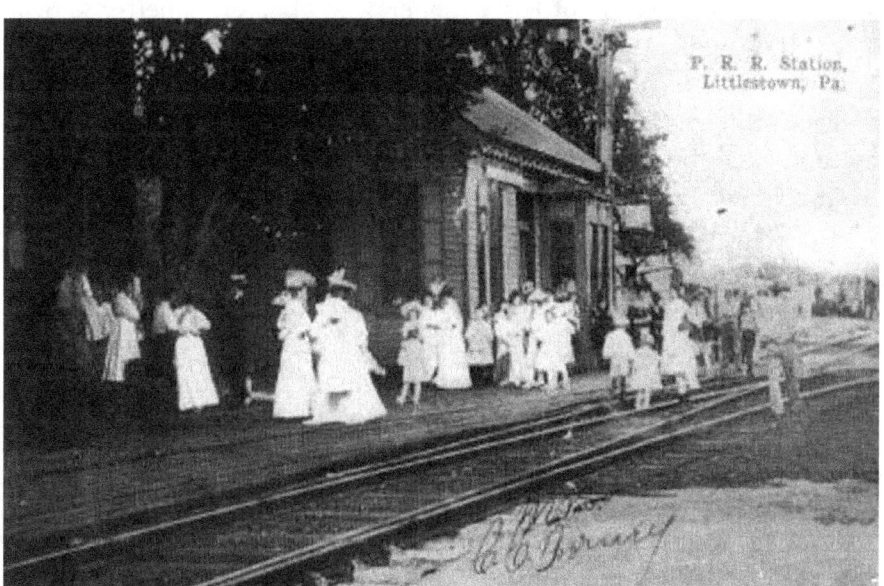

18-22: Littlestown, Pennsylvania

CHAPTER 19
Battles of Fort Wagner

Fort Wagner or **Battery Wagner** was a beachhead fortification on Morris Island, South Carolina, that covered the southern approach to Charleston Harbor. It was the site of two American Civil War battles in the campaign known as Operations Against the Defenses of Charleston in 1863, and was considered to be one of the toughest beachhead defenses constructed by the Confederate Army. Fort Wagner measured 250 by 100 yards and spanned an area between the Atlantic on the east and an impassable swamp on the west. Its walls, composed of sand and earth, rose 30 feet above the beach and were supported by palmetto logs and sandbags. The fort's arsenal included fourteen cannons, the largest a 10-inch (250 mm) Columbiad that fired a 128-pound shell. The fort fell only after a heavy bombardment, by Union gunboats, on September 7, 1863.

The First Battle of Fort Wagner, occurred on July 11, 1863. Only 12 Confederate soldiers were killed, as opposed to 339 losses for the U.S. side. The Second Battle of Fort Wagner, a week later, is better known. It was the Union attack on July 18, 1863, led by the 54th Massachusetts Volunteer Infantry, one of the first major American military units made up of black soldiers. Colonel Robert Gould Shaw led the 54th Massachusetts on foot while they charged, and was killed in the assault. Nearly 900 of these soldiers were wounded in this particular encounter.

The *Arago* was a wooden hulled, brig-rigged, sidewheel steamer built in 1855 by Westervelt & Sons at New York, New York. Chartered by the Union Army during the American Civil War for use as a troop transport and in operation with the South Atlantic Blockading Squadron throughout the war, *Arago* was the ship that returned the United States flag to Fort Sumter in April 1865. Returned to transatlantic passenger and freight service after the Civil War, she was sold to the Peruvian government in 1869.

On July 26, 1863 the *Arago*, filled to near capacity with wounded, sick, discharged and dead soldiers from the battles at Fort Wagner, including an ailing General George Crockett Strong,

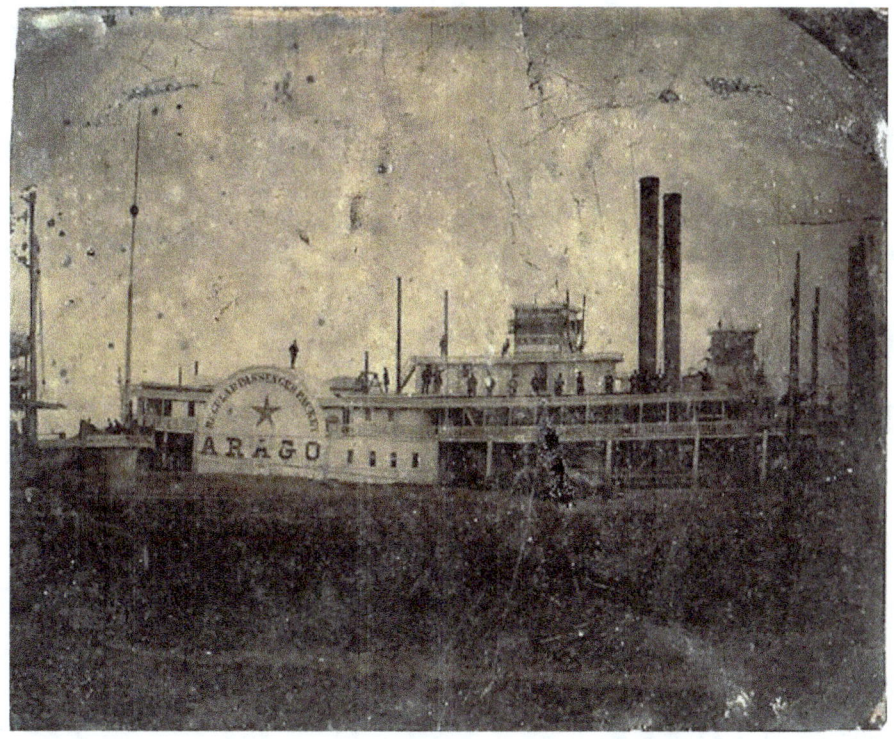

19-1: Hospital Transport Ship *Arago*

It is unsure where the *Arago* disembarked its wounded, however, it is possible that they were transported to hospitals located in New York, Washington, D.C. or Alexandria, Virginia.

CHAPTER 20
The Army of the Potomac

A network of general hospitals and hospital trains had established itself by the spring of 1864, when General Ulysses Grant prepared the Army of the Potomac to march toward Richmond, and General William Sherman was readying the Armies of the Cumberland, Ohio and Tennessee for the campaign through Georgia. In the upcoming campaign, the Army of the Cumberland would spearhead the entire effort. While both armies relied on railroads to evacuate their wounded, each army designed specialized hospital cars and used the hospital trains according to the dictates of the terrain and needs of the campaign.

For most of the Civil War (1862-1865), the portion of the Orange and Alexandria Railroad located in Fairfax County was under the control of the United States Military Railroad (USMRR). This fact would greatly enhance the ability of the Army of the Potomac in the upcoming campaigns against Richmond and Petersburg.

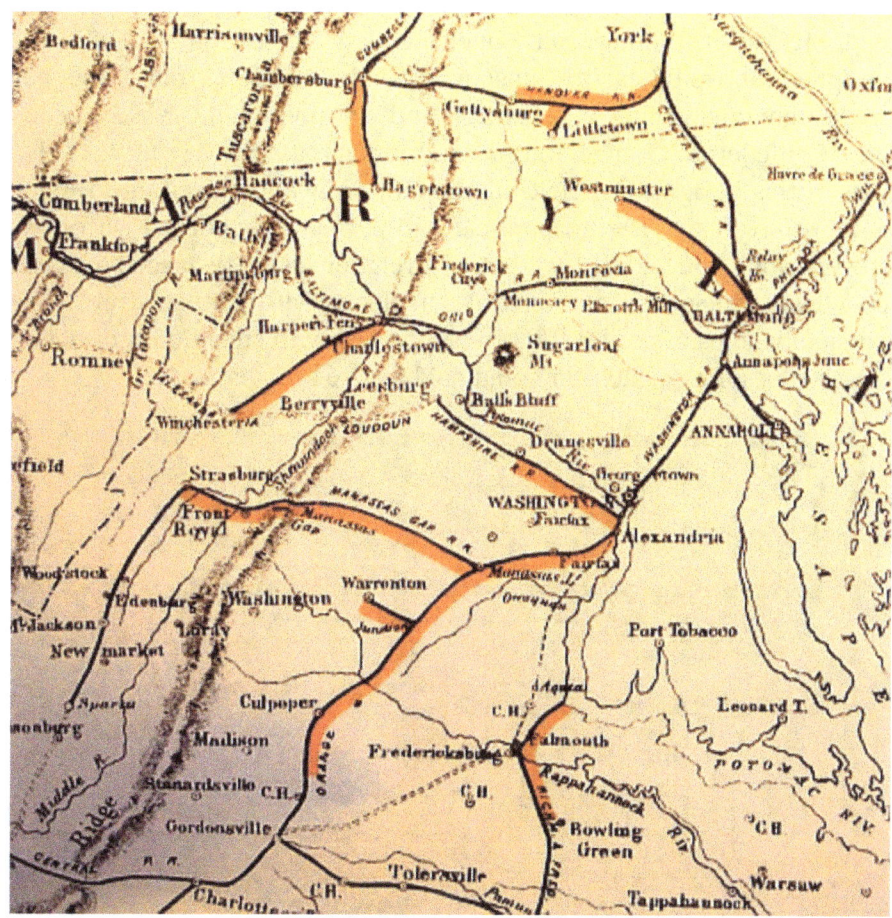

20-1: United States Military Railroad map

As General Grant prepared his campaign toward Richmond, Medical Director Thomas McParlin replaced Doctor Letterman in January 1864. McParlin, commissioned as Assistant Surgeon on March 31, 1849, was not as innovative as his predecessor, but he continued to refine the system Letterman established. In recognition of his attentive and efficient care of the soldiers of the Army of the Potomac, he was breveted the rank of Lieutenant Colonel on August 1, 1864.

In the Army of the Potomac, the complete hospital train consisted of twelve cars, ten cars for the sick and wounded, one for the kitchen and dispensary and one for the surgeon.

J. McCricket, the Assistant Superintendent of the Military Railroads, designed a hospital car to transport wounded soldiers from Culpepper to the general hospitals in Alexandria and Washington, D.C. via the occupied Confederate Orange and Alexandria Railroad. By May 1864, twelve cars of this design were built for the U.S. Army and placed into service within thirty days. The hospital car had permanent couches with mattresses along both sides. Two tiers of stretchers could be placed over the couches, suspended from vertical stanchions with leather straps. The outside handles of the litters were supported with steel hooks designed to serve as springs. Each car could hold fifty to sixty patients.

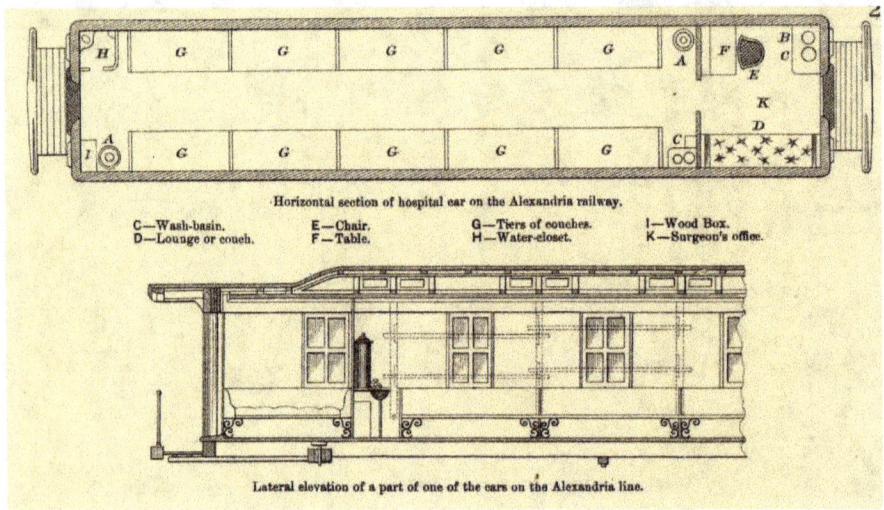

20-2: Lateral elevation of an Orange & Alexandria Railroad car

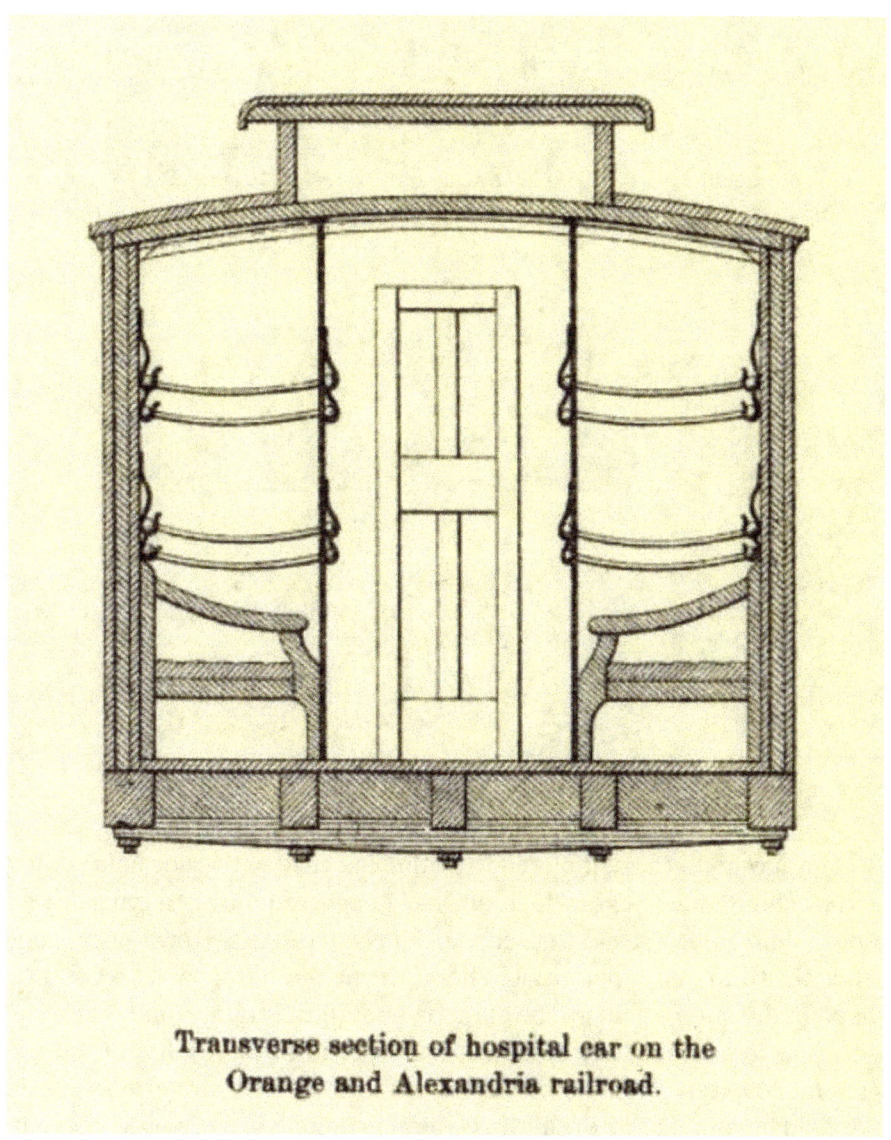

Transverse section of hospital car on the Orange and Alexandria railroad.

20-3: Transverse section of hospital car on the Orange & Alexandria Railroad

In support of this hospital car, McCrickett developed the kitchen and dispensary car.

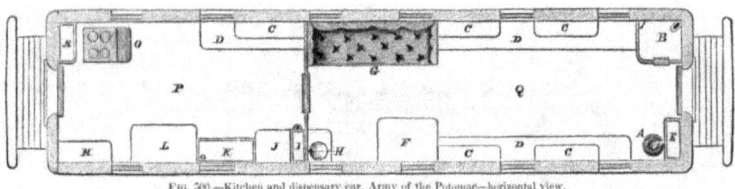

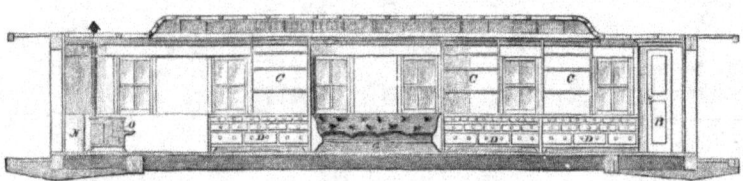

The kitchen and dispensary (FIGS. 500, 501) car was built according to plans prepared by the Assistant Superintendent of Military Railroads, J. McCrickett. The car was divided into two compartments. The dispensary contained a stove, A; a water-closet, B; cases for shelves, C; cases of drawers, D; wood-box, E; table or desk, F; couch, G; wash-basins, H. In the kitchen, P, were: C, cases of shelves; D, cases of drawers; I, water-cooler; J, refrigerator; K, sink for washing dishes; L, table; M, pantry; N, wood-box; O, cooking-stove.

20-4: McCrickett's kitchen and dispensary cars

The surgeon's car completed the train. Because of the normal swaying and pitching movements which normally occurred during a typical train ride at this point in time, surgeons normally did not perform operations while the train was in operation. Therefore, no operating tables were provided in the surgeon's car. The surgeon aboard the train would "stabilize" a patient in one of the hospital cars enroute until the train reached the general hospital. The surgeons either performed such surgery before (in the field hospital) or after (in the general hospital). If there was an emergency, I suspect they stopped and set up something outside.

The letters indicate: **A**, dispensary and steward's quarters; *a*, desk and book-case; *b*, shelves for medicines. This apartment contained also a revolving chair at the desk and a bed for the steward. **B**, surgeon's sitting-room; *d*, lounge;

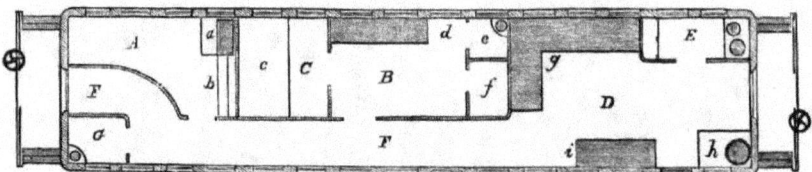

e, water-closet; *f*, clothes closet. **C**, surgeon's bedroom; *c*, bed. **D**, office; *g*, lounge; *h*, water-cooler; *i*, wood-box and stove. **E**, wash-room, with water basin, tank, and dressing

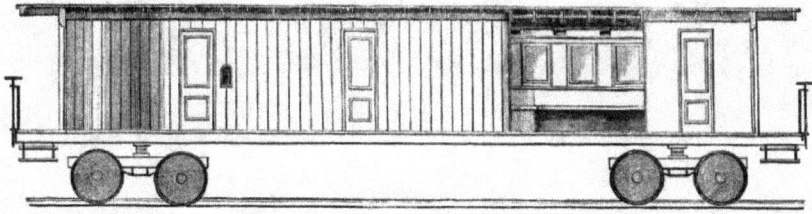

locker. **F F**, passage through car. **G**, water-closet.

20-5: Surgeon's car

The Army of the Potomac soon began to outrun its supply base in Culpepper, making it difficult to get supplies to the Army and wounded to the cities for medical care. In June 1864, General Grant established a new supply base at City Point, Virginia, located at the confluence of the James and Appomattox Rivers. He also located a 6,000-bed pavilion hospital that could, in emergencies, accommodate up to 10,000 men. The City Point & Army Railroad at City Point railroad line was constructed from the supply base to the front lines at Petersburg. By autumn, eighteen hospital trains ran daily between City Point and the front.

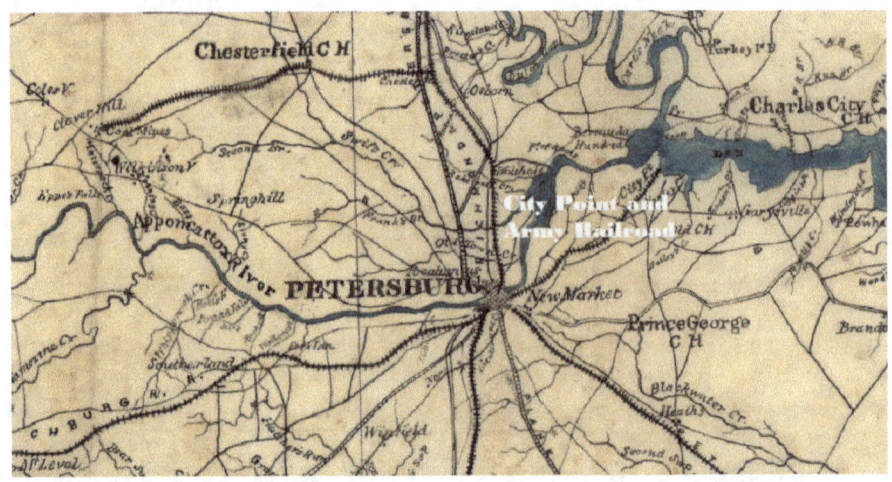

20-6: Petersburg

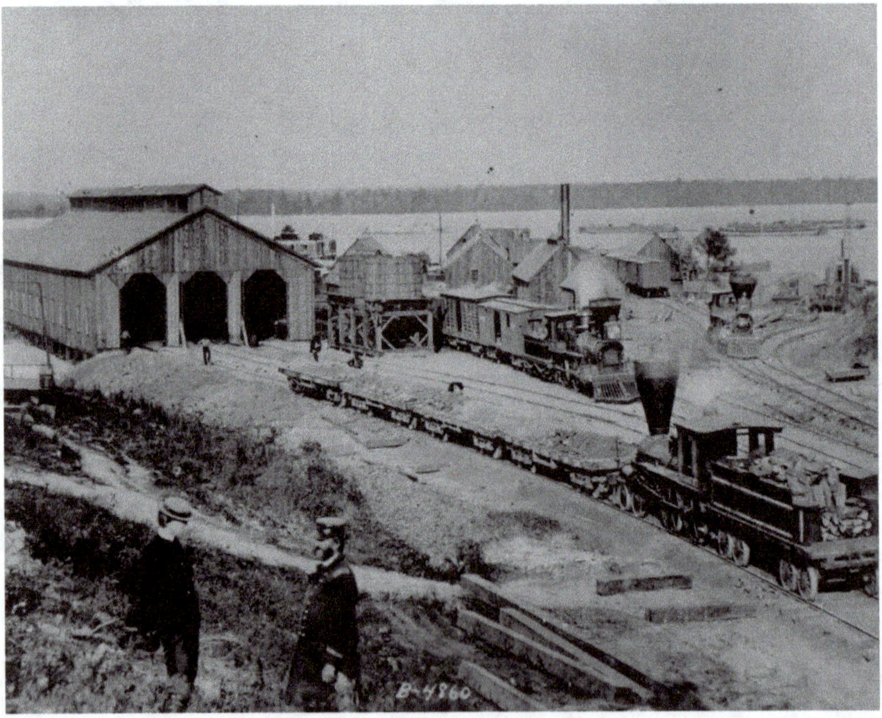

20-7: Depot of the U.S. Military Railroads, City Point, Virginia in 1864, showing the engine "President."

The hospital trains were often the improvised types typical of the earlier part of the war. Since the distance from Petersburg to City Point was about twenty miles and freight trains ran so frequently, getting the wounded to City Point was not a problem, but the way they were transported was. The boxcars which transported the wounded to City Point were sometimes packed with as many as twenty patients. In an attempt to dampen the harsh ride of the railcars to a tolerable level for severely wounded men, the floors of the cars were covered with a thick bed of fresh hay or straw and the patients were laid on overstuffed bed sacks. Once the train was underway, the hay on the floor quickly became matted down and dispersed, minimized its cushioning ability. After a heavy battle, it was difficult to get sufficient hay and dry leaves or pine boughs were sometimes substituted.

Adelaide Smith, an independent volunteer nurse at the City Point hospital, described the arrival of these trains:

> *"...from Petersburg front, sick and wounded were daily sent to the hospital, often on rough flat sand cars, over badly shaking tracks being brought as hastily as possible that they might receive proper care and help. The sight of these cars loaded with sufferers as they laid like logs, waiting their turn to be carried to the wards, -powder-stained, dust begrimed, in ragged torn and blood stained uniforms, with here and there a half severed limb dangling from a mutilated body, -was a gruesome, sickening one, never to be forgotten, and one which I tried not to see when unable to render assistance."*

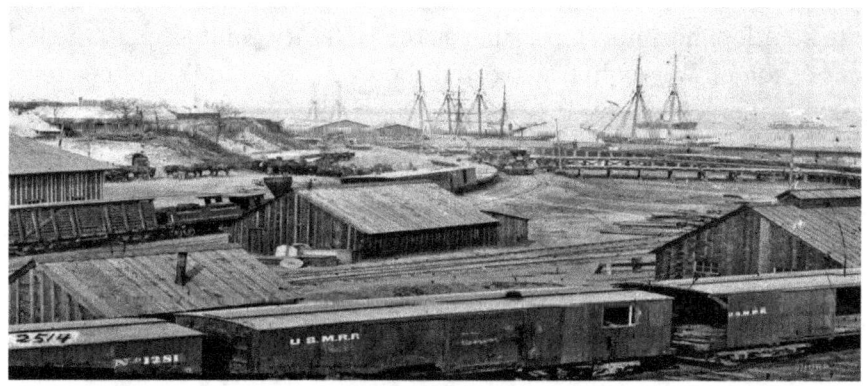

20-8: Harbor at City Point, Virginia

Once the wounded arrived they were taken to one of seven hospitals in City Point, the largest being the Depot Field Hospital. The sprawling 20 acre Depot Field Hospital served up to 10,000 patients. Twelve hundred tents, supplemented by ninety log barracks in the winter, comprised the compound, which included laundries, dispensaries, regular and special diet kitchens, dining halls, offices and other structures. Army surgeons administered the hospital aided by civilian agencies such as the United States Sanitary Commission and the U.S. Christian Commission.

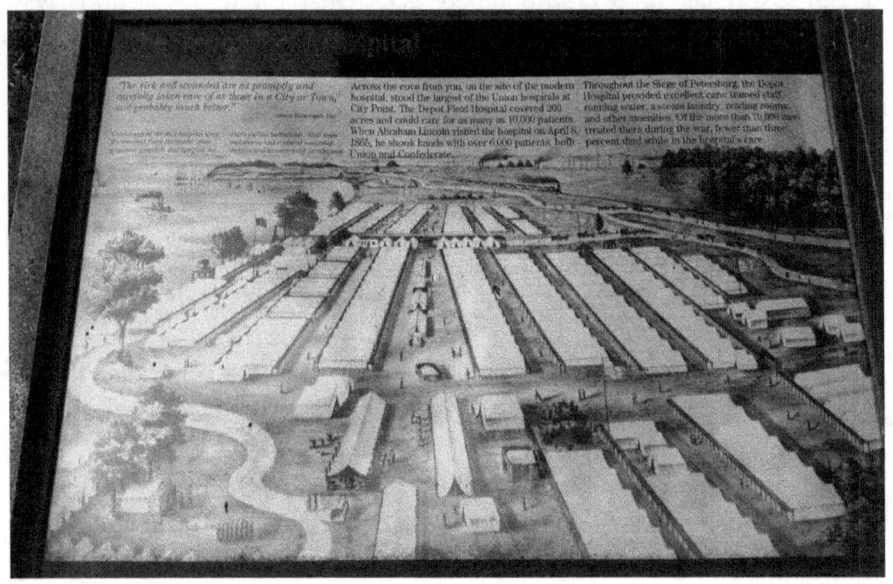

20-9: Depot Field Hospital at City Point

In addition, hospital ships, such as the USS *City Point* (seen in the left front of the photograph) transported the wounded, requiring long-term care, to general hospitals in New York City and Philadelphia.

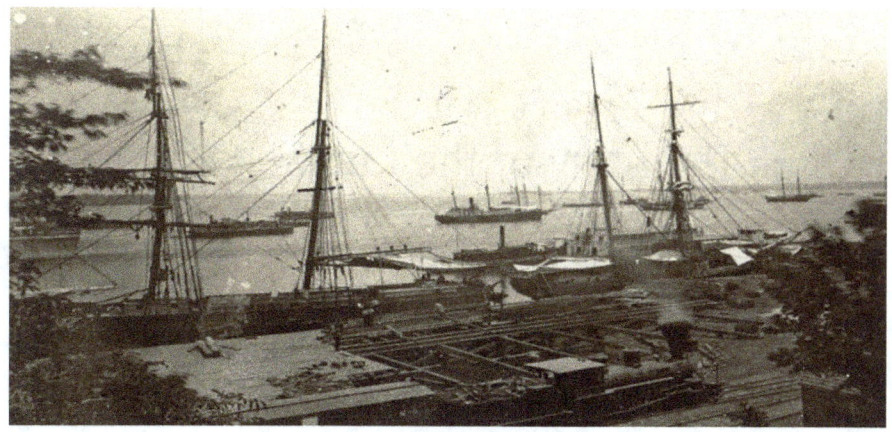

20-10: Hospital Transport Ship *City Point*

By January 1865, McParlin ordered specially built hospital railcars to be placed in service, greatly improving transportation of the wounded to City Point. These railcars were passenger cars configured to carry thirty patients in a design based on the Harris hospital car.

CHAPTER 21
The Army of the Cumberland

The Army of the Cumberland prepared its logistical medical support for the Atlanta Campaign well. It began to focus its sights on Atlanta beginning with the Battle of Chickamauga. In the fall of 1863, Acting Assistant Surgeon J. P. Barnum was tasked with outfitting a hospital train. He, according to Dr. F. L. Town, a Medical Inspector who examined the hospital trains, "had charge of the first hospital train built at Nashville. He studiously labored to improve and systematize its working, devised many expedients looking to the comfort of the patients in the days when the theory of hospital trains was not as well understood as now." The railcar designed by Barnum held thirty-three patients on litters hung from iron brackets by India-rubber springs. This concept was similar to the Harris car design.

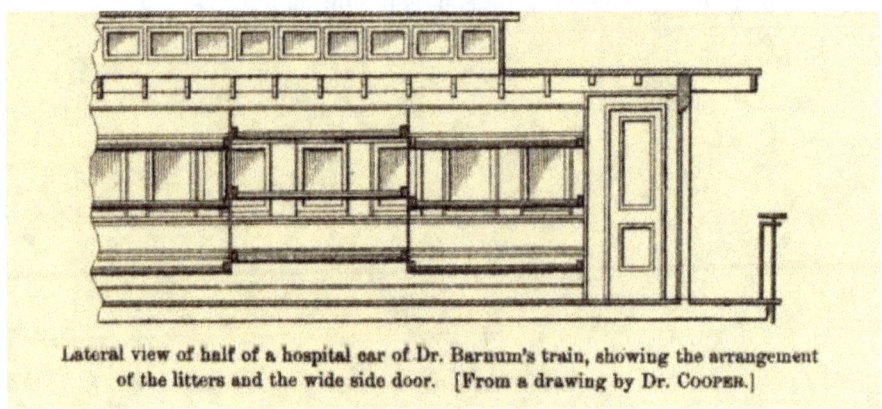

Lateral view of half of a hospital car of Dr. Barnum's train, showing the arrangement of the litters and the wide side door. [From a drawing by Dr. COOPER.]

21-1: Barnum's hospital train

Although the new Medical Director, Surgeon George Cooper, admired Barnum's enthusiasm and efficiency, he objected to his hospital car design, "... On the account of the surgeon being unable to manipulate the wounds, when they require dressing, without great inconvenience to himself. The space between the beds is too contracted, and that causes much complaint of the wounded. There is too much motion in the beds, and altogether the car is not a good one."

The Army of the Cumberland used hospital trains in order to evacuated the wounded to general hospitals in Nashville and Louisville. As the Army delved deeper and deeper into Georgia, beginning with the Battle of Chickamauga, it became more and more apparent that a new kind of hospital train had to be developed in order to care and feed the wounded. Taking care of up to two hundred wounded soldiers over such long distances was difficult. Delays were frequent, either due to immense supply trains headed to the front or from disruptions caused by confederate guerillas. Often the delay occurred at points where no rations could be drawn and no food could be prepared. As a result, a new kind of hospital train was indeed developed, one that could feed and care for a patient while en route as if he were in a general hospital. One observer wrote, "The conception of a complete hospital, with all of its appliances and means of comfort, propelled by steam, was first carried into practical operation in the medical department of the West, and its perfect success was most gratifying to all. In visiting these hospital trains, the air is found sweet and pure, the wards neat and inviting, and it may unhesitatingly be said that men on hospital trains are often as comfortable, and better fed and attended than many in permanent hospitals."

The configuration of the hospital train which was developed by the Army of the Cumberland was used on all of its runs during the Atlanta Campaign except for the following exceptions: The Doctor Elisha Harris hospital car, with its use of India rubber rings, was used on the Louisville and Nashville Railroad and the Nashville and Chattanooga Railroad runs, otherwise the hospital car design developed by Doctors Cooper and Herrick was used. These cars were fitted up under the immediate supervision of Medical Director Cooper, and of Surgeon Herrick, 34th Illinois volunteers. The rest of the consist and the specially designed locomotives remained the same throughout.

In 1863, Surgeon Robert O. Abbott, the Medical Director of the Department of Washington, ordered the construction of several complete hospital trains. Each train consisted of specially designed cars for the surgeon, the apothecary, a kitchen and ten ward cars. Variations of this design were used according to the logistical needs of the various armies. A typical hospital train, in operation during the Atlanta Campaign generally consisted of these cars: Surgeon's Car, Kitchen Car and a Hospital Car (up to five based on Doctors Cooper/Herrick design). A Baggage and Commissary Car, Passenger Car (soldiers that were not bedridden) and a Conductor's Car were also added as determined by the surgeon in charge of the train.

The Surgeon's Car was designed to lodge the surgeon in charge of the train and his hospital steward and provide accommodations for the dispensary of the train, with an office for the transaction of business. The surgeon and/or his steward had access to any of the hospital cars situated on either side of the Surgeon's Car in order to administer medication or in the event of an emergency.

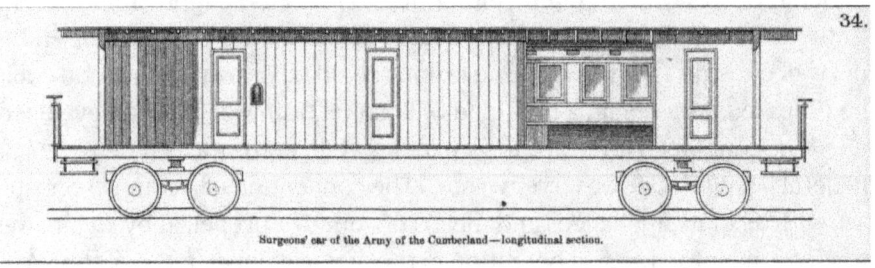

21-2: Surgeon's Car

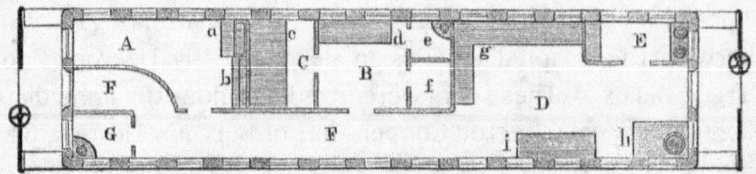

No. 1. *Surgeon's Car, Hospital Train of the Army of the Cumberland.*—This model represents an ordinary passenger car, with the seats removed, and with partitions and fixtures introduced, so as to lodge the surgeon in charge of the train and his hospital steward, and give accommodations for the dispensary of the train, with an office for the transaction of business.

FIG. 1.—*Horizontal plan of surgeon's car, Army of the Cumberland*

Figure 1 represents the arrangements of this car.

A, dispensary and steward's quarters; *a*, desk and book-case; *b*, shelves for medicines. This apartment contains also a revolving chair at the desk and a bed for the steward.

B, surgeon's sitting-room; *d*, lounge; *e*, water-closet; *f*, clothes-closet.

C, surgeon's bed-room; *c*, bed.

D, office; *g*, lounge; *h*, water-cooler; *i*, wood-box and stove.

E, wash-room, with water-basin, tank, and dressing locker.

F F, passage through car.

G, water-closet.

21-3: Cumberland Surgeon's Car

A fully equipped kitchen was capable of providing both meals and baked goods for the wounded. For those wounded confined to their litters in the hospital car(s), members of the U.S. Sanitary Commission both delivered and assisted these wounded with their meals. For those wounded, in the passenger car, which were not invalids and could walk with or without assistance, the kitchen car provided a dining room with a large table.

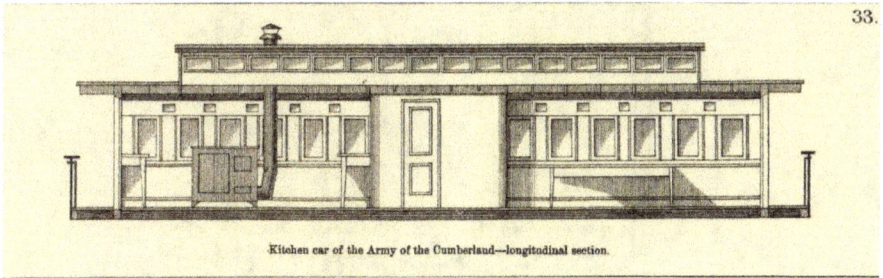

21-4: Kitchen Car

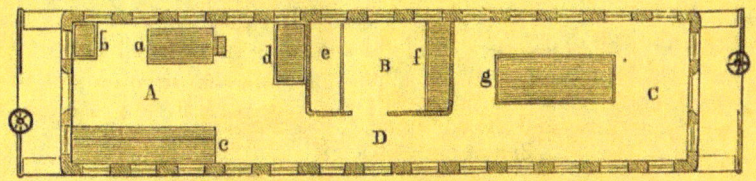

21-5: Kitchen Car

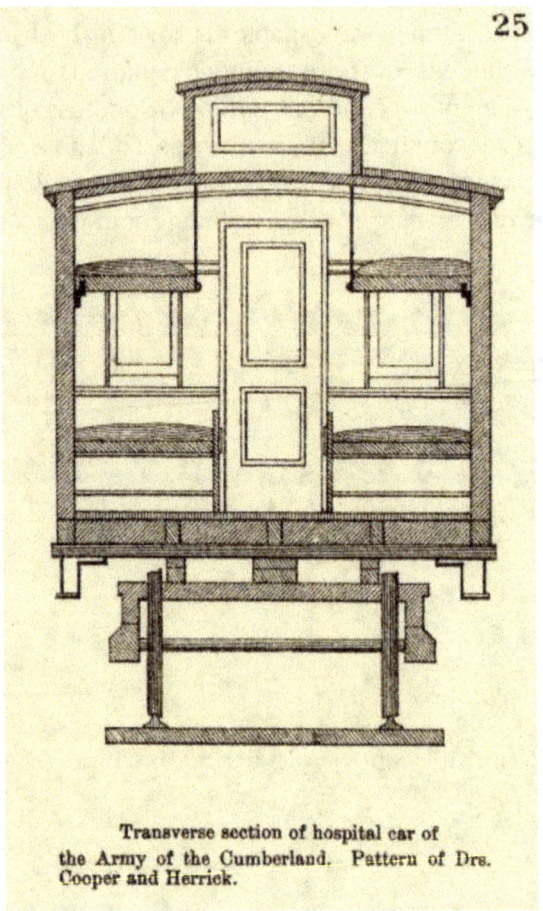

Transverse section of hospital car of the Army of the Cumberland. Pattern of Drs. Cooper and Herrick.

21-6: Cooper/Herrick Hospital Car

The beds inside the Cooper/Herrick designed hospital cars were arranged into two tiers. Wooden slats were placed over existing passenger seats, which had the seatbacks removed, to form the lower tier of beds. Mattresses were placed on the slats as a cushion. The upper tiers of beds were stretchers suspended from the ceiling by iron hooks. Eleven beds were thus formed on the lower tier and eleven beds formed on the upper level, so that the car could carry twenty-two patients. A six-foot wide doorway on one side of the car allowed ample space for carrying in of wounded soldiers on litters. Each car was provided with a water closet, stove, wood box and a water cooler.

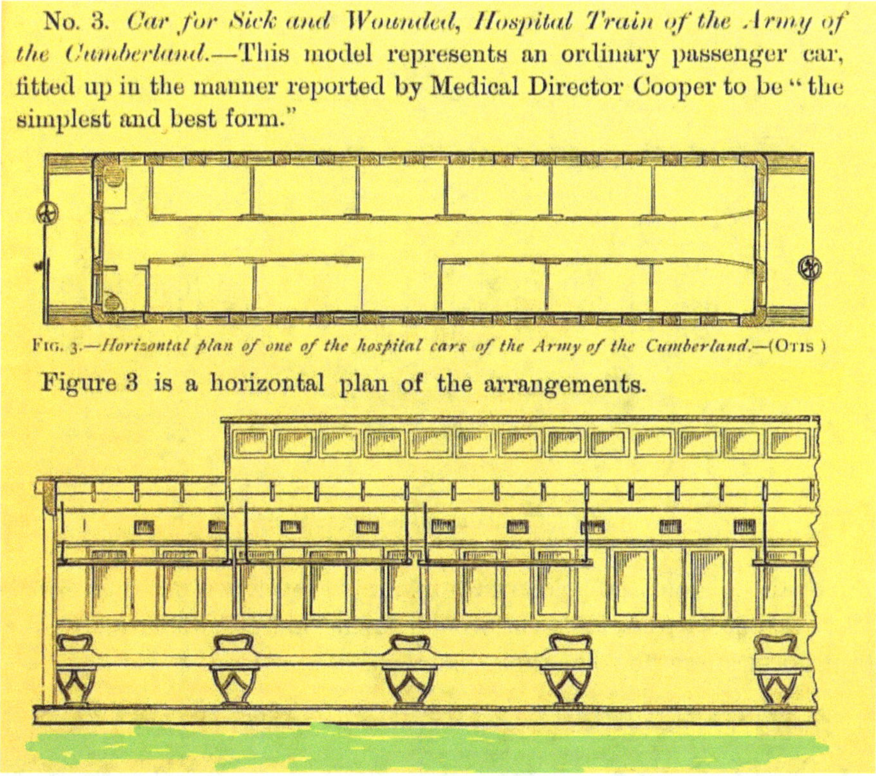

No. 3. *Car for Sick and Wounded, Hospital Train of the Army of the Cumberland.*—This model represents an ordinary passenger car, fitted up in the manner reported by Medical Director Cooper to be "the simplest and best form."

FIG. 3.—*Horizontal plan of one of the hospital cars of the Army of the Cumberland.*—(OTIS)

Figure 3 is a horizontal plan of the arrangements.

21-7: Cooper/Herrick Hospital Car

This car was used to store the baggage of the personnel on the train as well as the commissary stores of the train which included meat, coffee, sugar, flour, seasonings, vegetables, molasses, and so forth for the kitchen car, as well as soap, candles and other sundries. The large open space in the center was intended to carry barrels and large stores, such as flour and molasses. The two bunks were for the attendants belonging to the car.

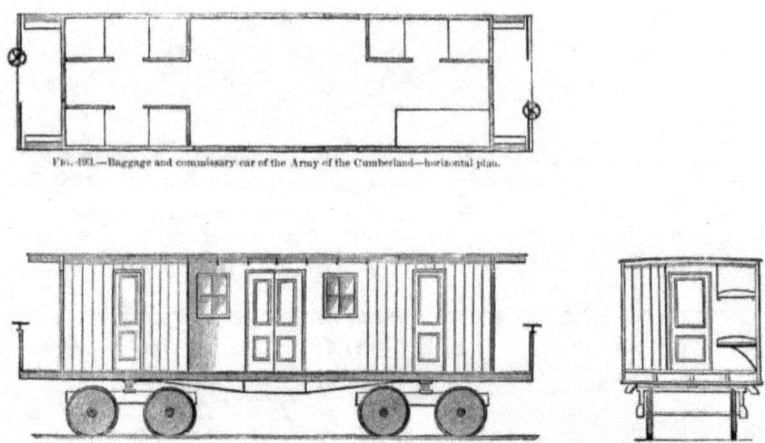

21-8: Cumberland Baggage Car

For those wounded soldiers who were seriously wounded and were fairly mobile, a passenger car would be the more suitable method of transportation rather than the hospital car.

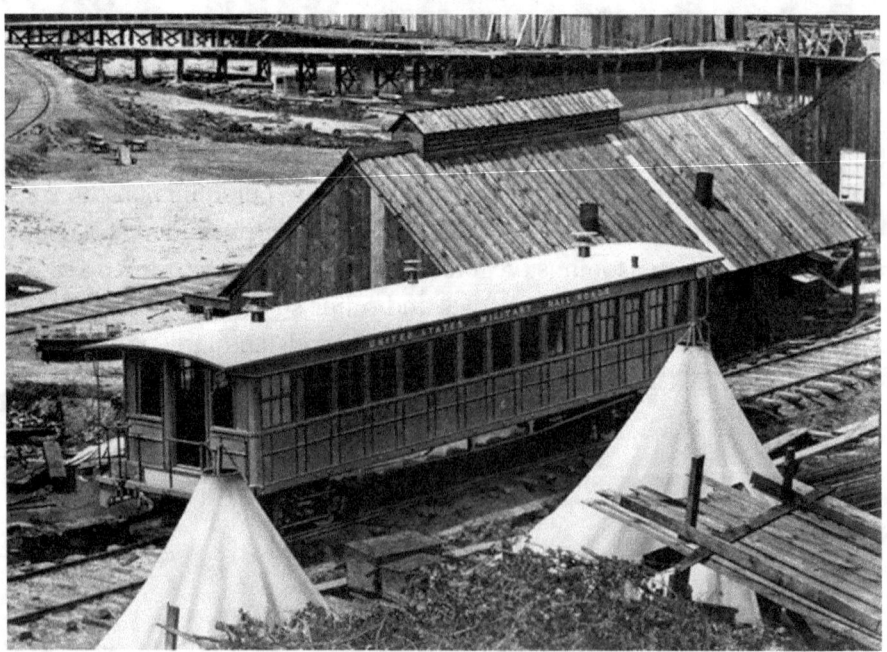

21-9: Cumberland Passenger Car

Cabooses had not entered the vocabulary yet but the need for a car for the crew was at the forefront. A unique car called the "way car" or "conductor's car" was showing up on many railroads. Many old images show this car as a converted house car. Amenities were few, but from the images we can see the caboose would soon be a reality.

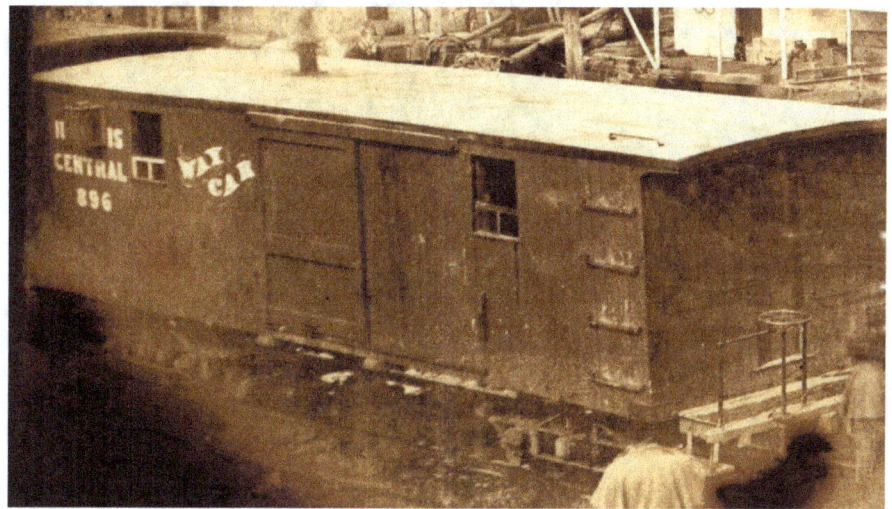

21-10: Cairo Waycar

The hospital trains were intentionally marked, in enormous red letters, "US HOSPITAL TRAIN" so as not to be fired upon by the enemy.

The locomotive leading the hospital train was intentionally painted a brilliant scarlet on the smokestack and the tender, with gold bands painted on the boiler, in order to clearly distinguish it from other trains. At night, three red lanterns were hung below the headlight to mark the train. These distinguishing signals were recognized by the Confederates, and the trains were never fired upon, or molested in any way. Doctor Cooper "was informed by wounded Confederate officers in Nashville, who were captured at the battle near that place, of the stringent orders given his troopers by Confederate Nathan Bedford Forrest not to interfere with hospital trains that were so certainly distinguishable from other trains. And, for the most part, it worked.

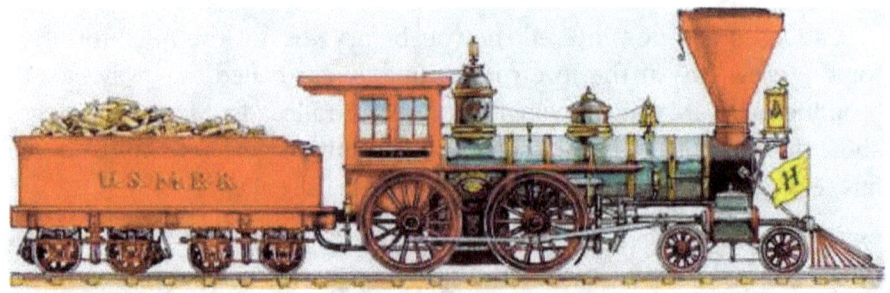

21-11: Engine "General Haupt"

The treatment of the wounded followed the Letterman system. Regimental aid stations evacuated the wounded soldiers to field hospital, located as close as possible, usually about two miles, to the front lines. The wounded then would be evacuated to a 1,000-bed depot hospital, intended to relieve the division field hospitals of their wounded within two to five days of injury. Once it had been determined that they could endure the trip, soldiers that were unlikely to be returned to their unit were sent by rail to the general hospitals in the rear. The wounded were gradually moved further and further to the rear, their beds filled by more recent casualties.

The Army of the Cumberland ran three hospital trains during the campaign, pulled by the best locomotives. A timetable was established to control the operation of these trains. One train ran from depot hospitals in Atlanta to Chattanooga, Tennessee. Another ran from Atlanta to Louisville, Kentucky and connected with a third train to Nashville, Tennessee. If necessary, a hospital car would be detached from one train and hooked to a connecting train without disturbing the patients. During the Atlanta Campaign, 25,184 wounded men made the twelve-hour journey to the general hospitals.

The hospital trains ran along rails not completely under the control of the U.S. Army. Although Confederate guerillas regularly harassed U.S. supply trains, they had orders to leave the hospital trains alone. On one occasion, enemy scouts stopped a hospital train directed by Assistant Surgeon Barnum and diverted it to a siding. After inquiring if there were sufficient stores on the train for the patients, they tore up the rails and ambushed the five subsequent supply trains that arrived at the point where the line had been torn up, leaving the hospital train alone to continue its journey.

CHAPTER 22
The Battle of Chickamauga

The Battle of Chickamauga was fought on September 18 - 20, 1863, between U.S. and Confederate forces and marked the end of the Union offensive in southeastern Tennessee and northwestern Georgia, the Chickamauga Campaign. It was the first major battle of the Civil War fought in Georgia and was the most significant Union defeat in the Western Theater. For the North and South, the battle involved the second-highest number of casualties of the entire war after the Battle of Gettysburg. The Union Army suffered 9,756 wounded in the aftermath of the battle.

The battle was fought between the Union Army of the Cumberland under Major General William Rosecrans and the Confederate Army of Tennessee under General Braxton Bragg, and was named for Chickamauga Creek, which meanders near the battle area in northwest Georgia and eventually flows into the Tennessee River about 3.5 miles northeast of downtown Chattanooga, Tennessee.

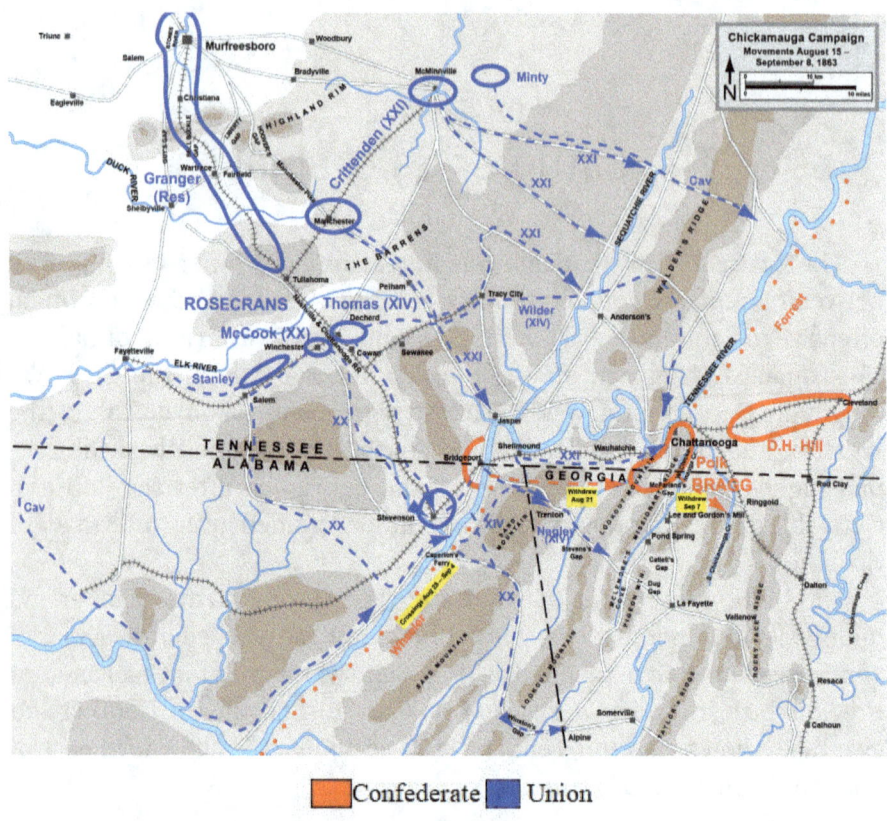

22-1: Chickamauga Campaign

A hospital train made up of one of the typical Army of the Cumberland specially designed locomotive and consist (including the Doctors Cooper and Herrick designed hospital cars) ran to Stevenson, Alabama after the Battle of Chickamauga in order to evacuate the half-starved wounded of that battle.

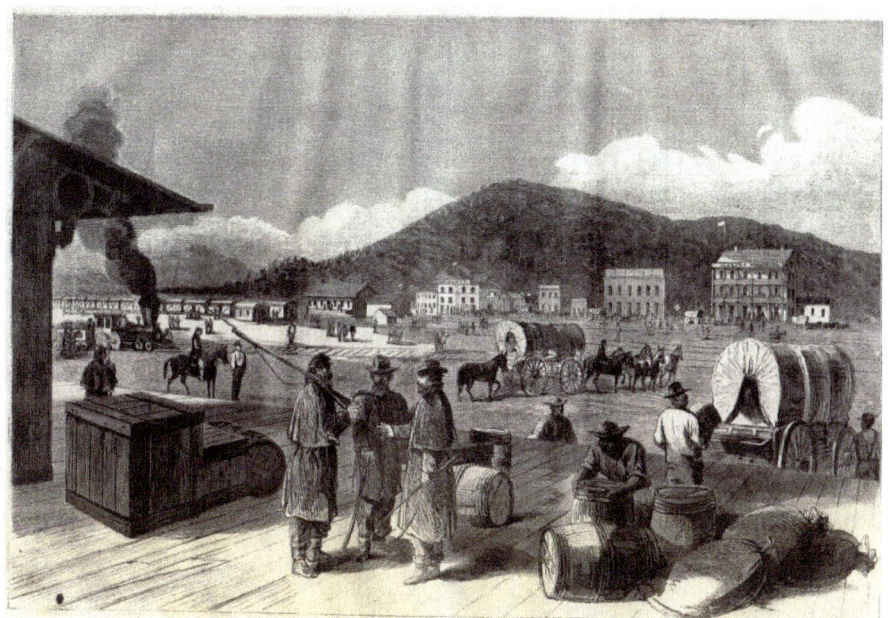

22-2: Stevenson, Alabama

CHAPTER 23
The Battle of Chattanooga

The Battle of Chattanooga began on November 24, 1863 when 70,000 Federal troops were amassed in the vicinity of the city of Chattanooga, Tennessee. The Federal breakout began with General George Thomas, Commander of the Army of the Cumberland, seizing Orchard Knob from the Confederates, and driving the Confederate line back. The next day, Joseph Hooker led the Federal attack at the Battle of Lookout Mountain, known as the "The Battle above the Clouds," and used his six-to-one advantage in men to defeat the Confederates.

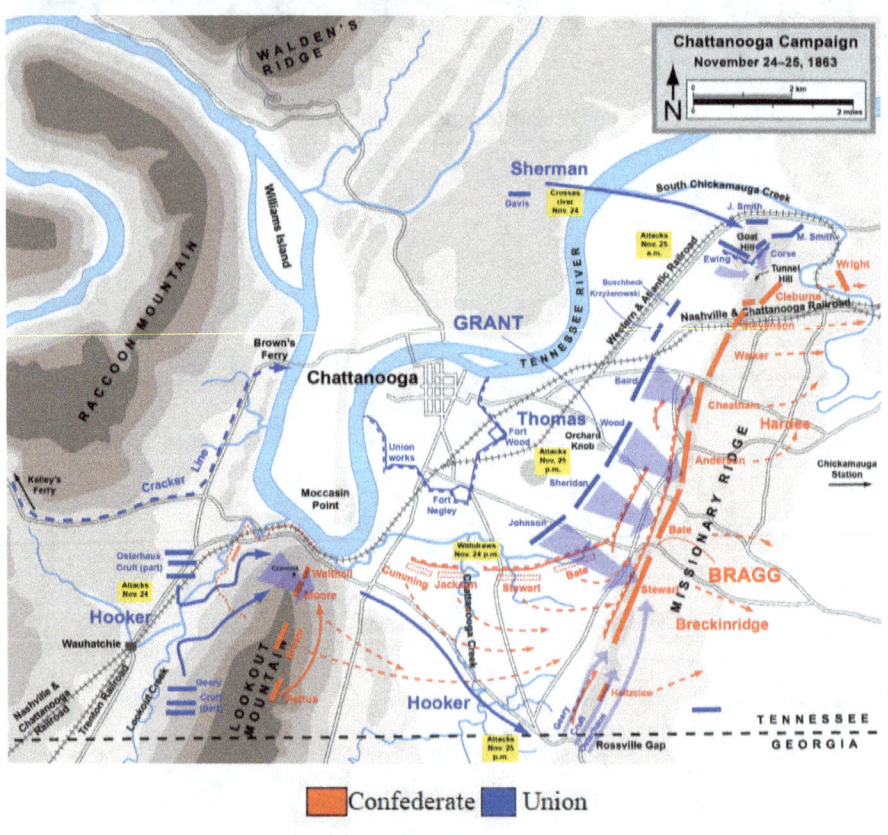

23-1: Chattanooga Campaign

These sketches were first printed in the *Harper's Weekly* publication of February 27, 1864. It depicts a Union hospital train, under the auspices of the Army of the Cumberland, crossing a railway bridge, along the Nashville and Chattanooga Railroad, on its run from Chattanooga to Nashville following the Battle of Chattanooga (November 24-25, 1863), as well as a view of the interior of a hospital car. The special hospital trains ran from Chattanooga to Nashville on a regular schedule, three times a week and continue through Sherman's Atlanta Campaign and his infamous March to the Sea. The locomotives of the hospital trains were painted red to identify them to roaming bands of Confederate guerillas, who usually, but not always let them pass. Stretchers were carried aboard and hung from straps; upon arrival in Nashville, the same stretchers were carried off. This arrangement made unnecessary the painful shifting of the wounded from stretcher to bed, and then again to stretcher. The sketches were done by Theodore R. Davis for the publication. Looking at the bottom sketch, the enlisted man on the right, next to the wash basin on its fluted stand, displays the sleeve insignia of a US Army hospital steward (though apparently reversed in this image): a green half chevron edged with yellow and bearing a yellow caduceus device. Note the Harris designed rubber bands secured at varying levels on the support posts, allowing the litters to shift in transit without touching the ones directly behind or in front of them. The *Harper's Weekly* article observed "Food of the most nourishing kind is furnished the wounded men, who, when they have arrived at their journey's end, are taken directly to the hospital upon the same stretchers which answer as couches upon the car. These beds are suspended from India-rubber bands attached to the frame-work of car, and, yielding to the slightest motion of the car, are as comfortable as the beds of the hospital."

The Harris designed hospital car was designed to hold three tiers of litters bunk-style along both side walls. The most severely wounded men were kept on the bottom tier.

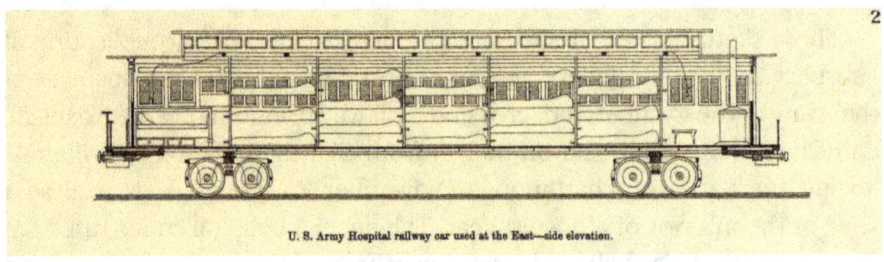

23-2: Harris Hospital Car

Except for the design of the hospital car, the configuration of the remainder of the hospital train was identical to the hospital train used by the Army of the Cumberland during the Atlanta Campaign.

In the book *Women's Work in the Civil War* by Dr. L.P. Brockett and Mrs. Mary C. Vaughan, here are the remarks of to one eyewitness who actually rode a hospital train from Chattanooga to Nashville entitled "ON A HOSPTAL TRAIN:"

> "I had the privilege of a ride on a hospital train from Chattanooga to Nashville, and an opportunity of seeing the plan of arrangement of the train. Imagine a car a little wider than the ordinary one, placed on springs, and having on each side three tiers of berths or cots, suspended by rubber bands. These cots are so arranged as to yield to the motion of the car, thereby avoiding that jolting experienced even on the smoothest and best kept road. I didn't stop to investigate the plan of the car then, for I saw before me, on either hand, a long line of soldiers, shot in almost every conceivable manner, their wounds fresh from the battle-field, and all were patient and quiet; not a groan or complaint escaped them, though I saw some faces twisted into strange contortions with the agony of their wounds. I commenced distributing my oranges right and left, but soon realized the smallness of my basket and the largeness of the demand, and sadly passed by all but the worst cases…
>
> "There were three hundred and fourteen sick and wounded men on board, occupying nine or ten cars, with the surgeon's car in the middle of the train. This car is divided into three compartments; at one end is the store-room where are kept the eatables and bedding, at the other, the kitchen; and between the two the

surgeon's room, containing his bed, secretary, and shelves and pigeonholes for instruments, medicines, etc. A narrow hall connects the store-room and kitchen, and great windows or openings in the opposite sides of the car give a pleasant draft of air. Sitting in a comfortable arm-chair, one would not wish a pleasanter mode of traveling, especially through the glorious mountains of East Tennessee, and further on, over the fragrant, fertile meadows, and the rolling hills and plains of Northern Alabama and middle Tennessee, clothed in their fresh green garments of new cotton and corn. This is all charming for a passenger, but a hospital train is a busy place for the surgeons and nurses.

"The men come on at evening, selected from the different hospitals, according to their ability to be moved, and after having had their tea, the wounds have to be freshly dressed. This takes till midnight, perhaps longer, and the surgeon must be on the watch continually, for on him falls the responsibility, not only of the welfare of the men, but of the safety of the train. There is a conductor and brakeman, and for them, too, there is no rest. Each finds enough to do as nurse or assistant. In the morning, after a breakfast of delicious coffee or tea, dried beef, dried peaches, soft bread, cheese, etc., the wounds have to be dressed a second time, and again in the afternoon, a third."

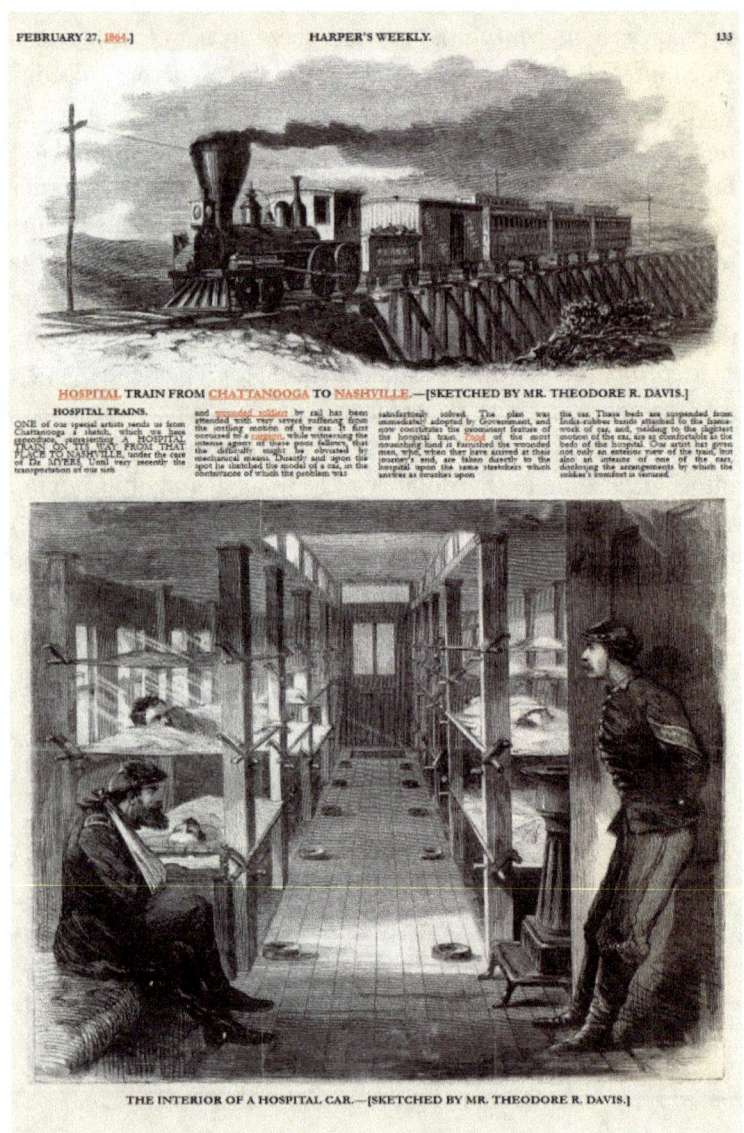

23-3: Hospital Train from Chattanooga to Nashville, Theodore R. Davis

CHAPTER 24
The Battle of Trevilian Station

The Battle of Trevilian Station (also called Trevilians) was fought on June 11–12, 1864 under the auspices of Union Lieutenant General Ulysses S. Grant's Overland Campaign against Confederate General Robert E. Lee's Army of Northern Virginia. During the course of the battle, Union cavalry under Major General Philip Sheridan fought against Confederate cavalry under Major Generals Wade Hampton and Fitzhugh Lee in the bloodiest and largest all-cavalry battle of the Civil War. The South incurred 813 casulties during the battle.

Sheridan's triple objective for his raid were to destroy stretches of the Virginia Central Railroad (VCR), provide a diversion that would occupy Confederate cavalry from understanding Grant's planned crossing of the James River, and to link up with the army of Major General David Hunter at Charlottesville. Hampton's cavalry beat Sheridan to the VCR at Trevilian Station and on June 11 they fought to a standstill. Brigadier General George A. Custer entered the Confederate rear area and captured Hampton's supply train, but soon became surrounded and had to fight desperately in order to avoid destruction.

On June 12, the cavalry forces clashed again to the northwest of Trevilian Station, and seven consecutive assaults by Brigadier General Alfred T. A. Torbert's Union division were repulsed resulting in heavy losses. Sheridan finally withdrew his force and rejoined Grant's army. The battle was a tactical victory for the Confederates and Sheridan failed to achieve his goal of permanently destroying the Virginia Central Railroad or of linking up with Hunter. Its distraction, however, may have contributed to Grant's successful crossing of the James River.

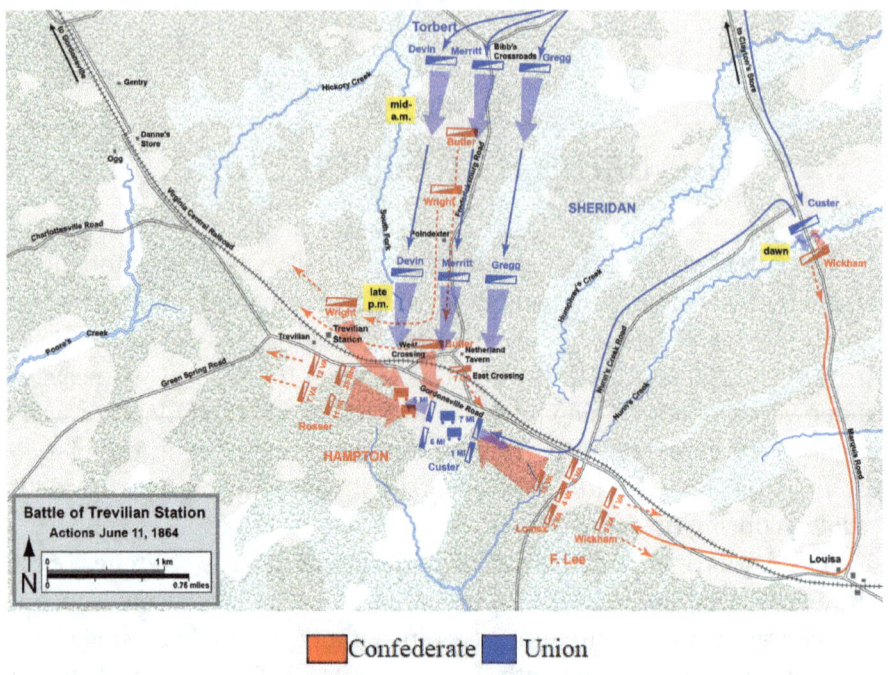

24-1: Trevilian Station

The wounded Confederate soldiers from the Battle of Trevilian Station were transported via the Virginia Central Railroad to Gordonsville first the Gordonsville Depot and then to the Gordonsville Receiving Hospital.

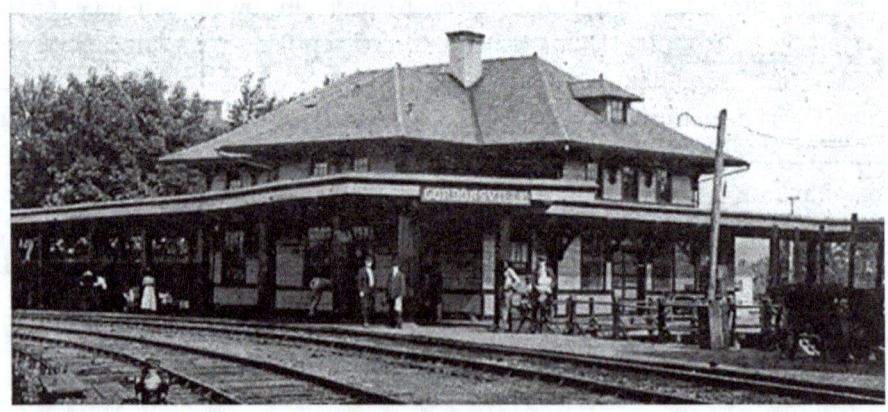

24-2: Gordonsville Depot

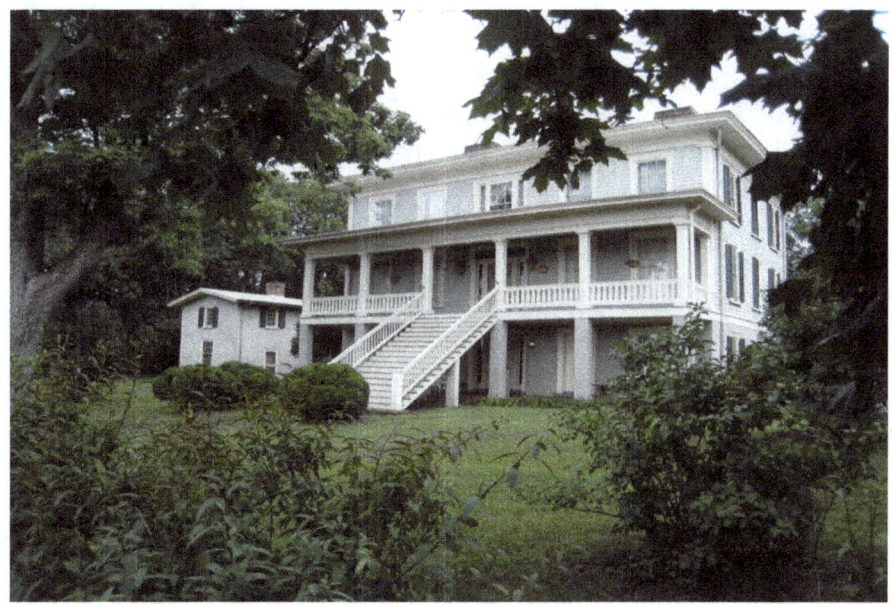

24-3: Exchange Hotel

In March 1862, the Exchange Hotel, in Gordonsville, Virginia, was taken over by military authorities and received the wounded from the battlefields for the duration of the war. It became known as the Gordonsville Receiving Hospital. Dr. B.M Lebby of South Carolina was the director and its operation continued under his leadership until October 1865. Although this was primarily a Confederate facility, the hospital treated the wounded from both sides. Twenty-six Union soldiers died here.

CHAPTER 25
The Atlanta Campaign

A network of general hospitals and hospital trains had established itself by the spring of 1864, when General William Sherman was readying the Armies of the Cumberland, Ohio and Tennessee for the campaign through Georgia.

The Atlanta Campaign was a series of battles fought throughout northwest Georgia and the area around Atlanta during the summer of 1864. Union Major General William Tecumseh Sherman as head of the Military Division of the Mississippi, which in fact, entailed command of all Union troops in the Western Theater of the war (Army of the Cumberland, Army of the Ohio and the Army of the Tennessee), invaded Georgia from the vicinity of Chattanooga, Tennessee, beginning in May 1864, and was opposed by the forces under Confederate General Joseph E. Johnston. Johnston's Army of Tennessee withdrew toward Atlanta in the face of successive flanking maneuvers by Sherman's group of armies. In July, the Confederate President, Jefferson Davis, replaced Johnston with the more aggressive General John Bell Hood, who began challenging the Union Army in a series of costly frontal assaults. Hood's army was eventually besieged in Atlanta and the city fell on September 2, shortly after the fall of Jonesboro on August 31, setting the stage for Sherman's March to the Sea which hastened the end of the war. The Union incurred 22,822 wounded during this campaign while 18,952 Confederate soldiers were wounded.

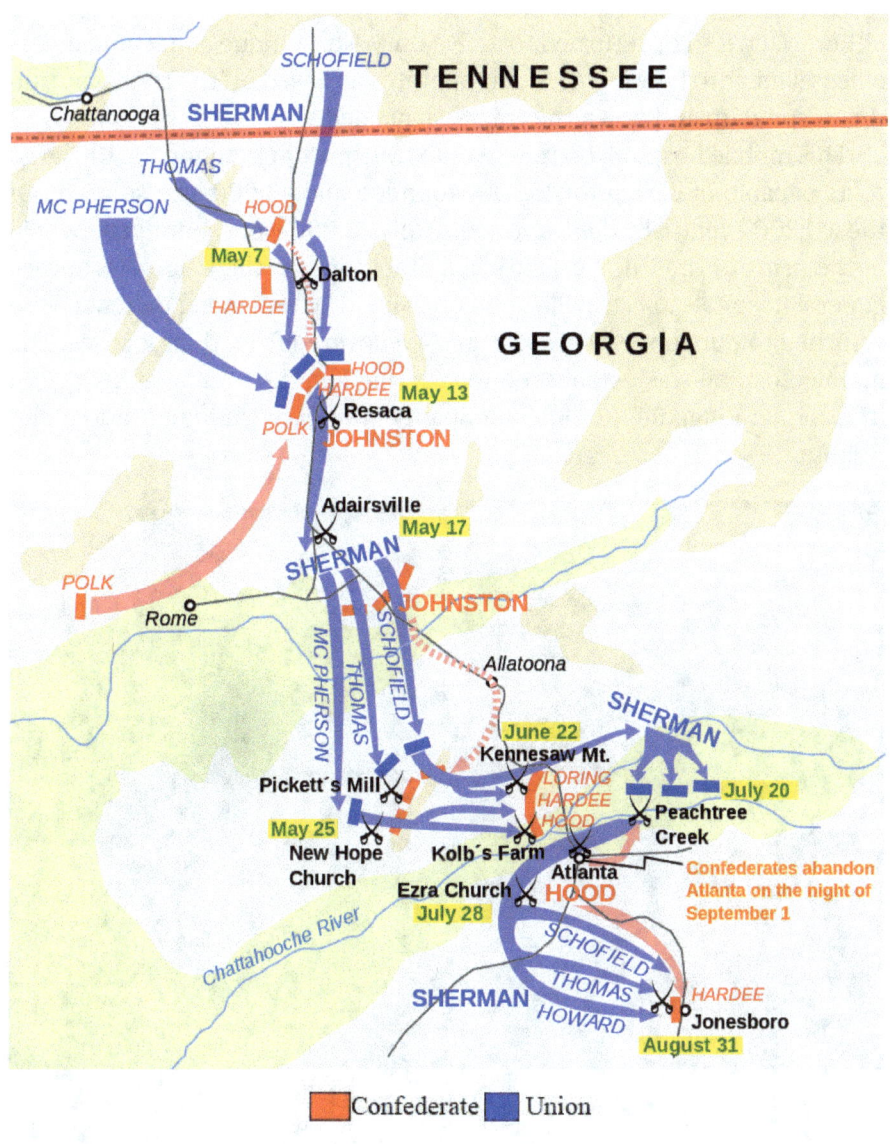

25-1: The Atlanta Campaign

During the 1864 Atlanta Campaign, the Union Army of the Cumberland conceived of a landmark approach in the handling and transportation of the sick and wounded called a "Travelling General Hospital." It literally followed the army down the captured Confederate Western and Atlantic (W&A) Railroad keeping all the sick and wounded together until they were either evacuated or returned to active duty. This unique concept in medicine is similar to how a MASH unit operates all based off the trains moving the hospital up and down the tracks as needed.

This mobile hospital, on rails, would transport in freight cars, 100 large tents capable of caring for 15,500 wounded and 43,000 sick soldiers. Of these 1,200 eventually died, approximately 26,000 were sent north by rail, in the Army of the Cumberland's hospital trains, to the longer-term care general hospitals in Nashville and Louisville. The remaining patients were returned to duty once they sufficiently recovered from their injuries. The mobile hospital was established for varying lengths of time at six places in Georgia: Ringgold, Resaca, Big Shanty, Marietta, Vining's Station, and Atlanta.

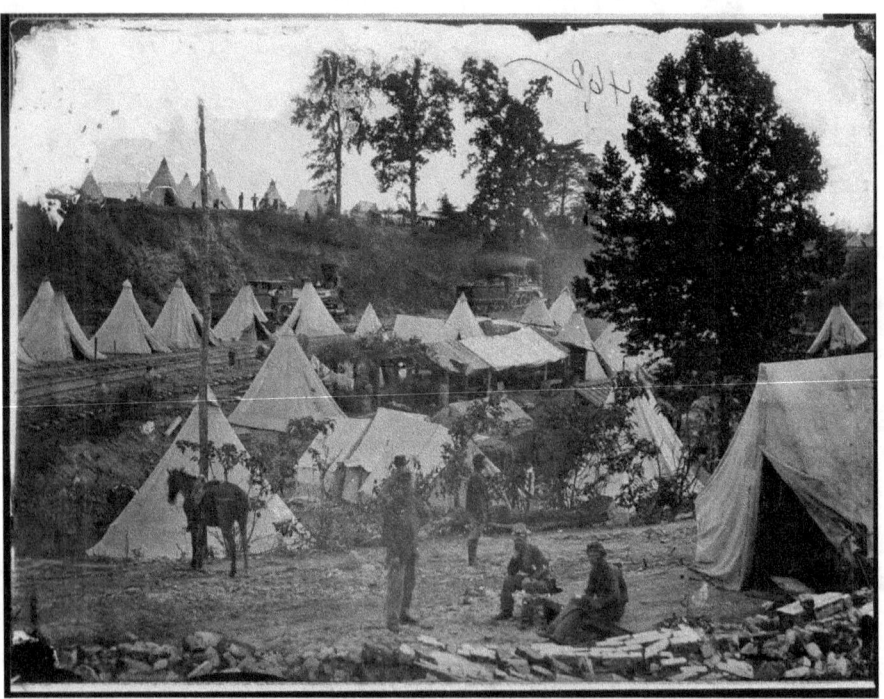

25-2: Field Hospital at City Point, Virginia

The systematic evacuations of the wounded by railroad were probably the most interesting medical feature of the entire Atlanta Campaign.

The Western and Atlantic (W&A) Railroad was used to evacuate wounded Union soldiers to Chattanooga. The Army of the Cumberland then used the Nashville and Chattanooga Railroad to transport these wounded soldiers, on a regular schedule three times a week, from Chattanooga to general hospitals located in Nashville which included The Old Gun Factory, University Building and Ensley Buildings.

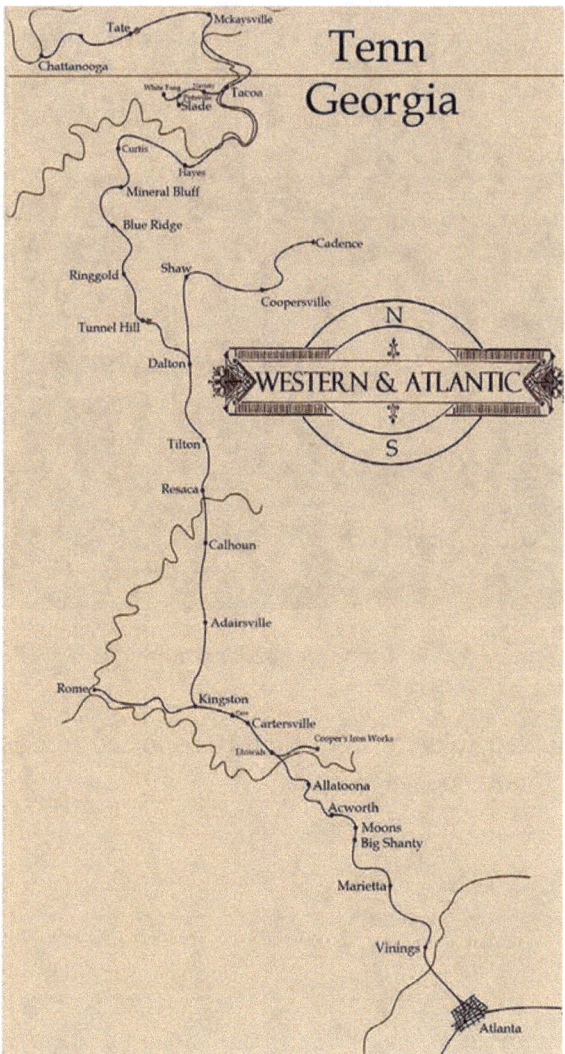

25-3: Western & Atlantic Railroad map

Wounded Union soldiers were transported by rail via the W&A Railroad to the Chattanooga Union Station more commonly known as the Union

Depot in Chattanooga. It was constructed between the years 1857-1859. It was jointly owned and operated by the W&A Railroad and the Nashville and Chattanooga Railroad.

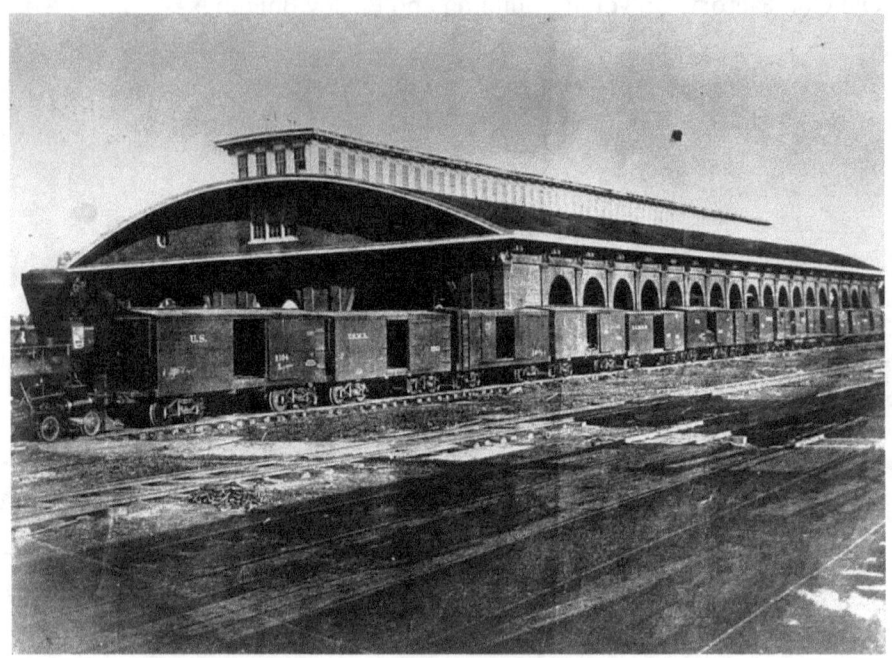

25-4: Union Depot, Chattanooga

These wounded soldiers were then transported to Nashville via the Nashville and Chattanooga Railroad.

The Atlanta Campaign | 185

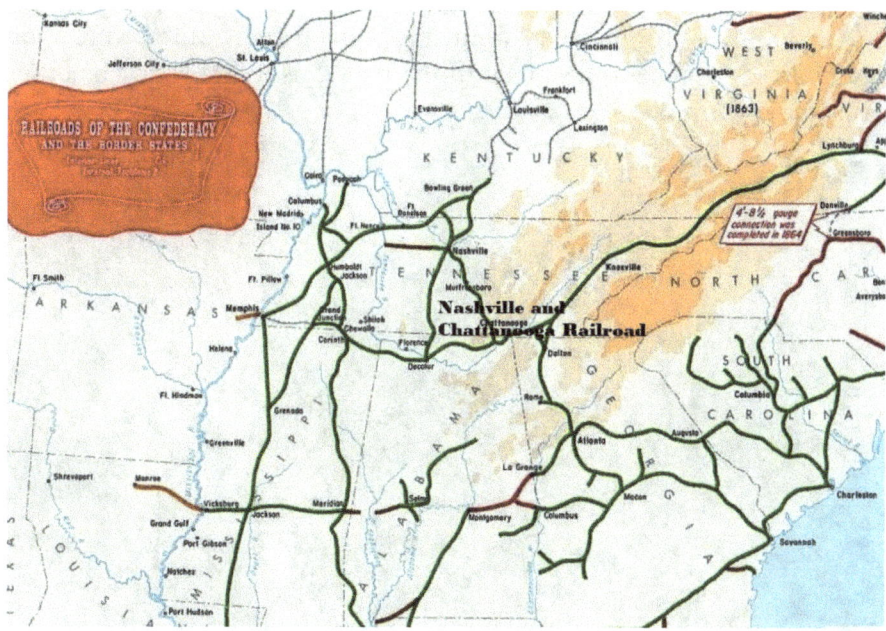

25-5: Nashville & Chattanooga Railroad

These wounded soldiers would have arrived at the Nashville and Chattanooga Railroad Depot.

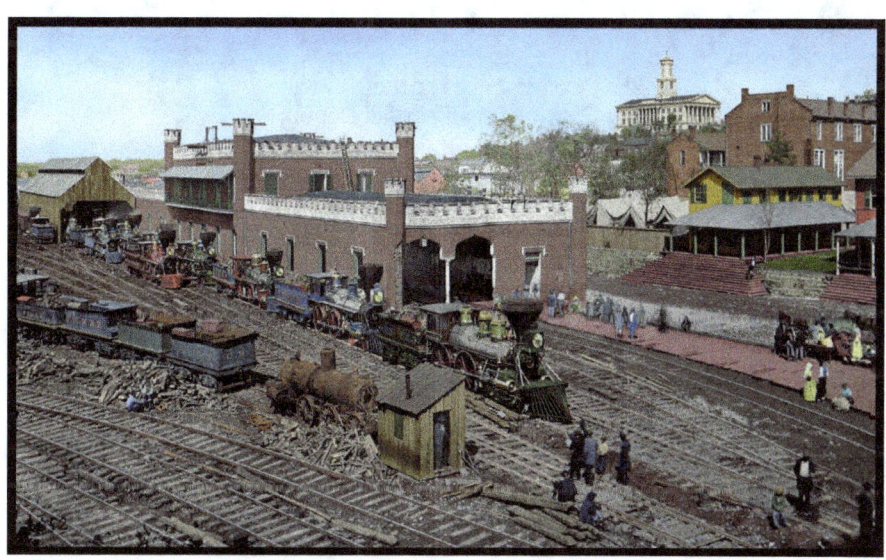

25-6: Nashville & Chattanooga Railroad Depot

Once they were unloaded from the hospital trains, they were then transported to general hospitals throughout Nashville by cart or other available conveyance.

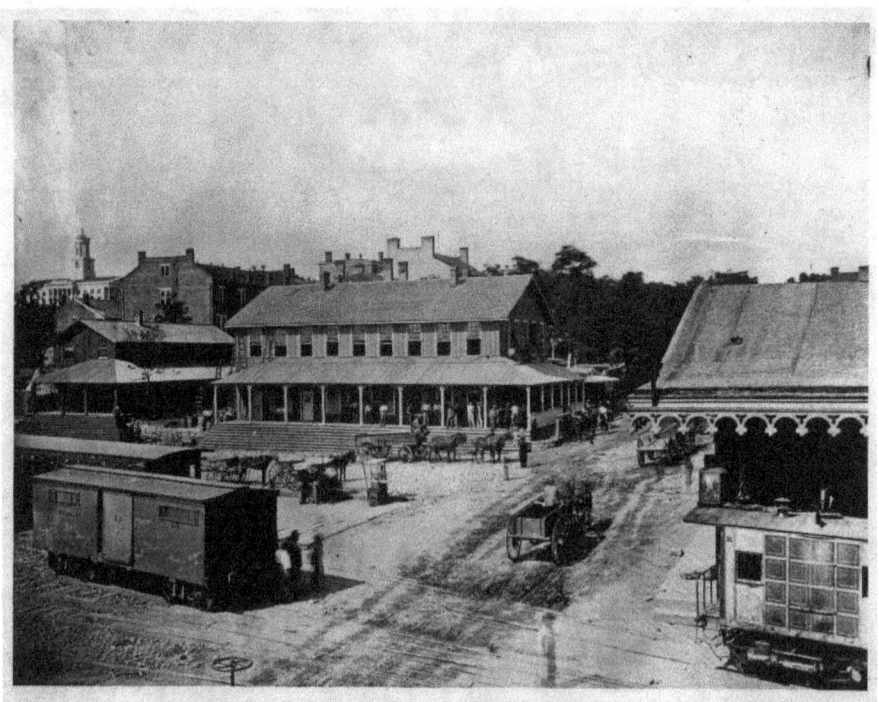

25-7: Conveyances at the Nashville & Chattanooga Railroad Depot

In addition, once these wounded arrived in Nashville, they could also be transported to hospitals in Louisville, Kentucky via the Louisville and Nashville Railroad.

On the other side of the battle lines, wounded Confederate soldiers were hastily evacuated from Atlanta hospitals, on the brink of the city's imminent surrender to Sherman's Army, and brought to Atlanta's Union Station, also known as Union Depot. The Station would be burned on or around November 11, 1864, along with all Confederate railroad rolling stock, by Union troops under Sherman's direction. In addition, all surrounding tracks are torn up, heated by bonfires, and bent into so-called bowties around telegraph poles.

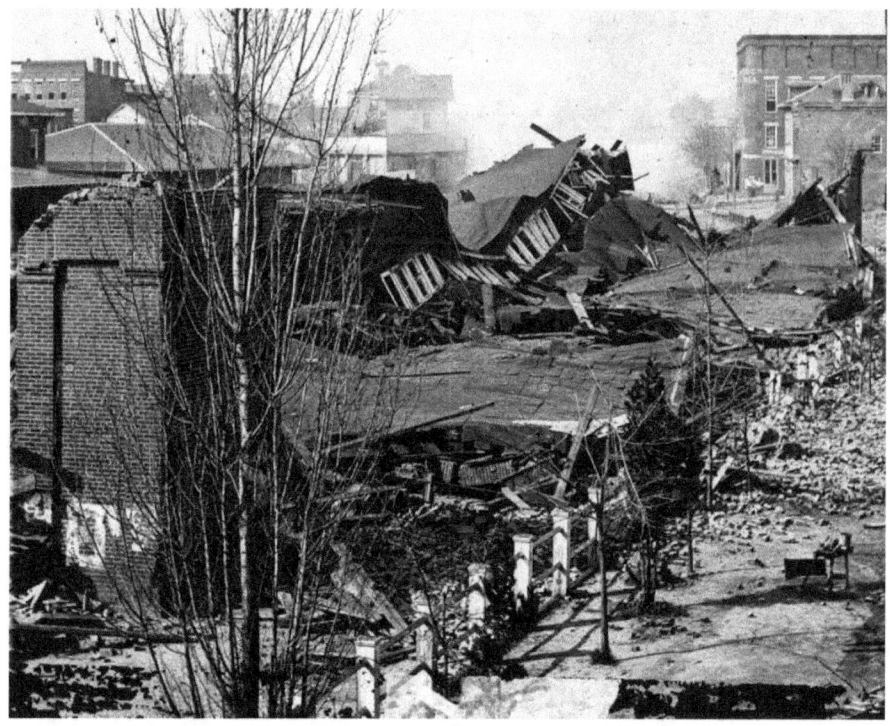

25-8: Destruction of Atlanta's Union Station

The wounded Confederate soldiers were quickly loaded onto any available rail cars for their journey out of the city. After being medically stabilized for their journey, their trip began with little provision made for their creature comfort.

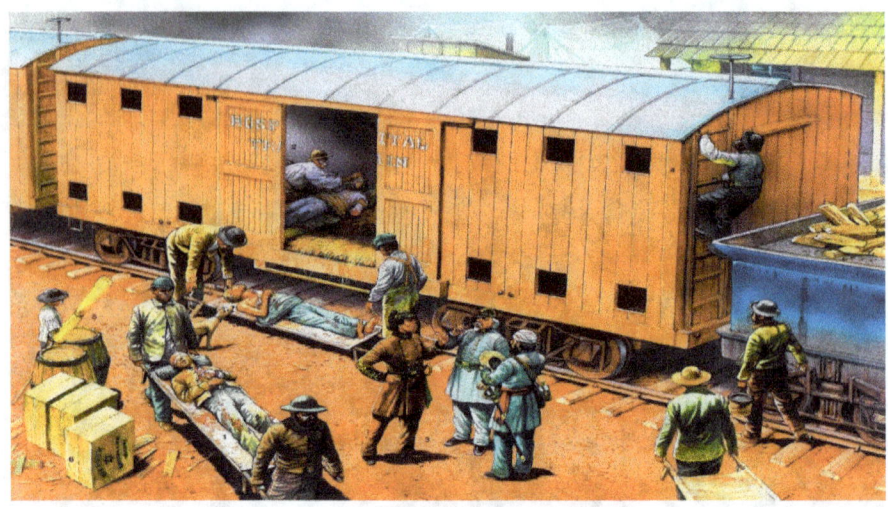

25-9: Confederate Hospital Train

The man in charge of coordinating the all the medical aspects of the Confederacy, during the war, was Doctor Samuel Hollingsworth Stout. He was born in Tennessee and served as the organizer and medical director of the Hospital Department of the Confederate Army in Tennessee, Mississippi, Georgia, Alabama, and Louisiana.

During the Battle of Chickamauga, Doctor Stout noticed that someone under his command had placed the wounded in commissary wagons filled to the brim with pine-tops and covered with a blanket; as it turned out, this simple improvement on the straw method provided a more comfortable way of evacuating the wounded than anything offered by the latest technology in wagon springs. The wounded soldier was tucked into the nest of straw, pine-tops, prairie grass or whatever soft material the staff could gather locally. Stout had discovered that the sprung horse drawn ambulance wagons bounced the patient around agonizingly; applying the principle to the railroad, Stout got rid of all his "so-called railway ambulance cars" with their tiered berths, being used regularly by the Virginia Central Railroad, and replaced them with boxcars complete with one or two feet of straw on the floor. Stout reasoned that not only did the soldiers in the top berths have to breathe the rank air expelled by the sick and wounded on the lower berths, but the train's jolting knocked the top tiers around painfully and sometimes even threw men from their bunks. Placing the wounded on the floor kept them at the car's center of gravity and gave them an easier ride. Doctor Stout's simpler yet more comfortable ambulance car, using straw rather than slung litter/bunks, featured ventilation holes cut near the roof and the floor. In this case a baggage car, coupled directly to the tender, has also been modified to evacuate wounded soldiers.

African-American men frequently served as ambulance-drivers and litter-bearers in the Confederate army. During various battles a significant number of black men working as teamsters for the Quartermaster Department were shifted to ambulance duty, transporting the wounded to waiting trains at wayside stations. In addition to caring for the patients and supplying water, the nurses on board ambulance cars changed out the bedding, cleaned the car, and kept it stocked with fresh bandages. Patients also had to be fed; but while Civil War doctors knew that a proper diet was essential to health, they had an appallingly poor understanding of the causes of disease and infection. One Confederate doctor noted after the war that it was fortunate that he eventually ran out of sponges and had to resort to rags, since the sponges were loaded with germs that spread from one patient to the next. Two medical officers - an assistant surgeon ranking as captain and a surgeon ranking as major - confer with an infantry officer. Although Confederate uniforms were extremely varied, there is plenty of evidence to show that Confederate doctors at least tried to keep themselves properly outfitted. One surgeon mentioned in a letter to his wife that while he had an officer's uniform the only material he could get was brown; his brigade later issued gray cloth for the officers, but there was not enough to go round, so they had to draw lots for it. Doctors were frequently left behind to care for the severely wounded, which meant inevitable capture; wishing to be recognizable as non-combatants, they made sure that they had their identifying green sashes. In the days before automatic brakes and couplers the brakemen held the most dangerous job on the train. In peace and wartime alike they frequently fell to their deaths, and the trainmen who had to join cars with the old link-and-pin couplers often had a few fingers missing. Each wagon had its own brake, and the brakeman had to climb up to the roof of baggage cars to turn the brake wheel by hand. Confederate surgeons were also expected to carry yellow hospital flags and red ambulance flags, and to display them conspicuously for easy identification. As in the North, numerous charitable organizations across South contributed to the war effort. Matron Kate Cumming often received food packages for her patients and staff from the Hebrew Military Aid Society based in her adopted hometown of

Mobile, Alabama. The aid society packages often included spices, wines, preserves, oysters, and sardines; clothing and money were also donated to help the patients.

Following the Battles of Atlanta and Jonesboro, General Hood hastily evacuated his wounded using the only railroad still operating at the time, the Macon and Western Railroad southeast to the Army of the Tennessee hospitals along its route, including Griffin, Milner, Barnesville, Vineville, Forsyth, and Macon. Unfortunately, a number of these often temporary hospitals had to be subsequently evacuated and relocated as Sherman's moved south-southeastward on its infamous "March to the Sea" to Savannah beginning on November 16, 1864.

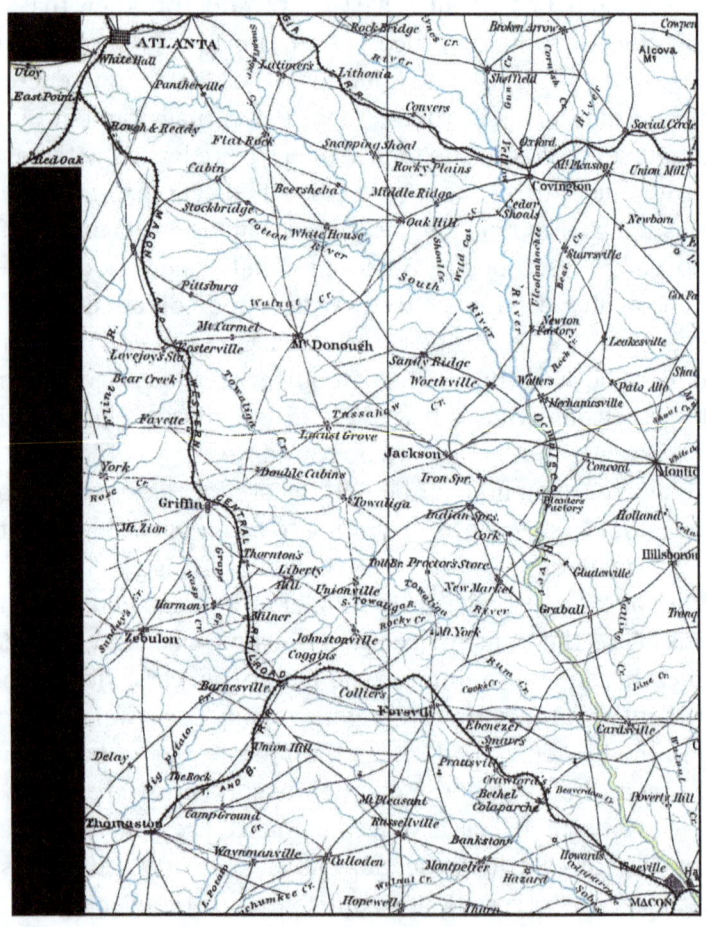

25-10: Map of the Macon and Western Railroad in southeastern Georgia

Mobile, Alabama. The aid society packages often included spices, wines, preserves, oysters, and sardines; clothing and money were also donated to help the patients.

Following the Battles of Atlanta and Jonesboro, General Hood hastily evacuated his wounded using the only railroad still operating at the time, the Macon and Western Railroad southeast to the Army of the Tennessee hospitals along its route, including Griffin, Milner, Barnesville, Vineville, Forsyth, and Macon. Unfortunately, a number of these often temporary hospitals had to be subsequently evacuated and relocated as Sherman's moved south-southeastward on its infamous "March to the Sea" to Savannah beginning on November 16, 1864.

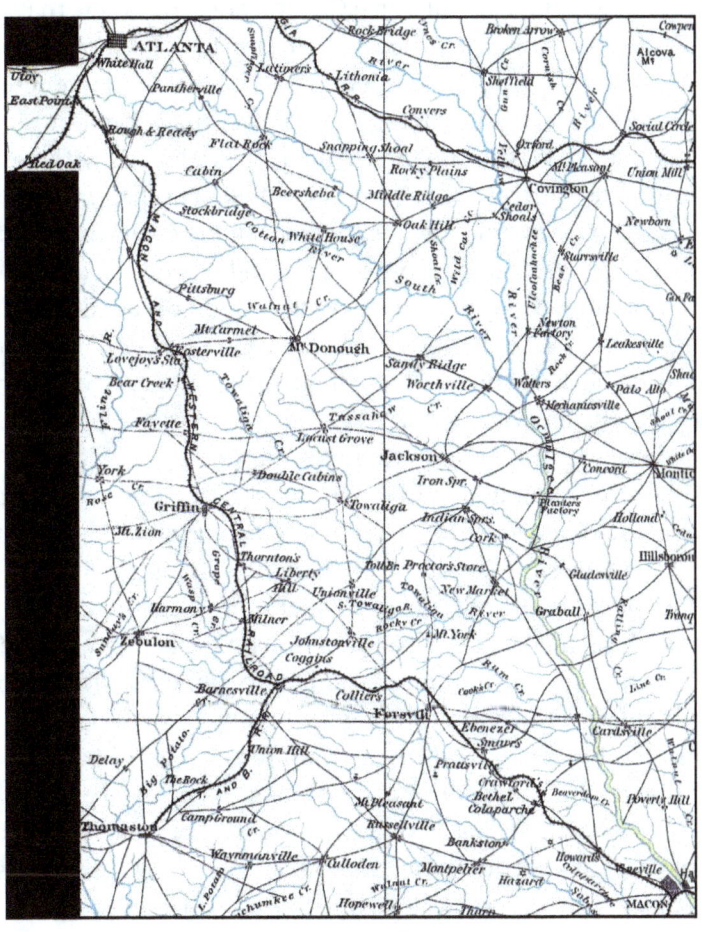

25-10: Map of the Macon and Western
Railroad in southeastern Georgia

ier ride. Doctor Stout's simpler yet more comfortable ambulance car, using straw rather than slung litter/bunks, featured ventilation holes cut near the roof and the floor. In this case a baggage car, coupled directly to the tender, has also been modified to evacuate wounded soldiers.

African-American men frequently served as ambulance-drivers and litter-bearers in the Confederate army. During various battles a significant number of black men working as teamsters for the Quartermaster Department were shifted to ambulance duty, transporting the wounded to waiting trains at wayside stations. In addition to caring for the patients and supplying water, the nurses on board ambulance cars changed out the bedding, cleaned the car, and kept it stocked with fresh bandages. Patients also had to be fed; but while Civil War doctors knew that a proper diet was essential to health, they had an appallingly poor understanding of the causes of disease and infection. One Confederate doctor noted after the war that it was fortunate that he eventually ran out of sponges and had to resort to rags, since the sponges were loaded with germs that spread from one patient to the next. Two medical officers - an assistant surgeon ranking as captain and a surgeon ranking as major - confer with an infantry officer. Although Confederate uniforms were extremely varied, there is plenty of evidence to show that Confederate doctors at least tried to keep themselves properly outfitted. One surgeon mentioned in a letter to his wife that while he had an officer's uniform the only material he could get was brown; his brigade later issued gray cloth for the officers, but there was not enough to go round, so they had to draw lots for it. Doctors were frequently left behind to care for the severely wounded, which meant inevitable capture; wishing to be recognizable as non-combatants, they made sure that they had their identifying green sashes. In the days before automatic brakes and couplers the brakemen held the most dangerous job on the train. In peace and wartime alike they frequently fell to their deaths, and the trainmen who had to join cars with the old link-and-pin couplers often had a few fingers missing. Each wagon had its own brake, and the brakeman had to climb up to the roof of baggage cars to turn the brake wheel by hand. Confederate surgeons were also expected to carry yellow hospital flags and red ambulance flags, and to display them conspicuously for easy identification. As in the North, numerous charitable organizations across South contributed to the war effort. Matron Kate Cumming often received food packages for her patients and staff from the Hebrew Military Aid Society based in her adopted hometown of

As General Sherman began his advance on Savannah from Atlanta, Confederate General Hood moved his remaining forces southeast away from the city. As he retreated, the Confederate Army of Tennessee established a complex network of mobile hospitals, along the way in advance of Sherman's Army. As enemy forces approached, Doctor Stout literally packed up everything from the senior surgeons to the forks and spoons and sent the entire complement by train (or occasionally by horse and wagon) to a safer location. Stout had established certain criteria for hospital sites. The town had to be on the Macon and Western Central Railroad because trains were the quickest and most comfortable way to transport large numbers of patients. It also needed to have plenty of water and wood, appropriate buildings with empty land for hospital expansion, and adequate food available in the area. The town should also be some distance from battlefields and the risk of raids. Unlike the general hospitals of Virginia, which stayed in one place, the Army of Tennessee hospitals went through waves of movement due to military conditions. Most hospital movements occurred in the summer of 1863, before the Battle of Chickamauga; around December 1863, after the Battle of Chattanooga; during the Atlanta campaign in the summer of 1864; and during and after John Bell Hood's Tennessee campaign in the fall and winter of 1864.

During the Atlanta campaign, especially, hospitals were continually relocating, even into Alabama, to avoid raiders from Union General William T. Sherman's army. At its peak during the summer of 1864, Stout's hospital system had at least fifty hospitals in nineteen Georgia towns, but locations changed frequently. In the fall of 1864 the hospitals tried to follow Hood into Tennessee, but due to deteriorating and indirect transportation routes, most were waylaid in Alabama or Mississippi and never provided any help to the sick and wounded.

After they returned from the Tennessee campaign, Stout's hospitals were reestablished in dozens of locations in Georgia locations, but they were very short on supplies. Although some of the hospitals were ordered to Charlotte, North Carolina, in April 1865, they were unable to go because of transportation collapse. Instead, most hospitals in Georgia surrendered when captured by Union forces, though some continued to serve needy soldiers traveling home.

The Army of Tennessee hospitals were located at one time or another in each of the following Georgia cities and towns: Adairsville, Albany, Americus, Athens, Atlanta, Augusta, Barnesville, Calhoun, Cassville,

Catoosa Springs, Cherokee Springs, Columbus, Covington, Cuthbert, Dalton, Eatonton, Forsyth, Fort Gaines, Fort Valley, Geneva, Greensboro, Griffin, Kingston, LaGrange, Macon, Madison, Marietta, Milledgeville, Milner, Newnan, Palmetto, Resaca, Ringgold, Rome, Thomaston, Tunnel Hill, Vineville, and West Point.

CHAPTER 26
The Battle of Nashville

The Battle of Nashville was a two-day battle during the so-called Franklin-Nashville Campaign and represented the end of large-scale fighting west of the coastal states in the Civil War. The battle was fought near and around Nashville, Tennessee, on December 15-16, 1864, between the Confederate Army of Tennessee under Lieutenant General John Bell Hood and Federal forces under Major General George H. Thomas. In one of the largest victories achieved by the Union Army during the war, Thomas attacked and routed Hood's army, largely destroying it as an effective fighting force for the remainder of the war. The Union forces suffered a total of 2,558 wounded as a result of the battle.

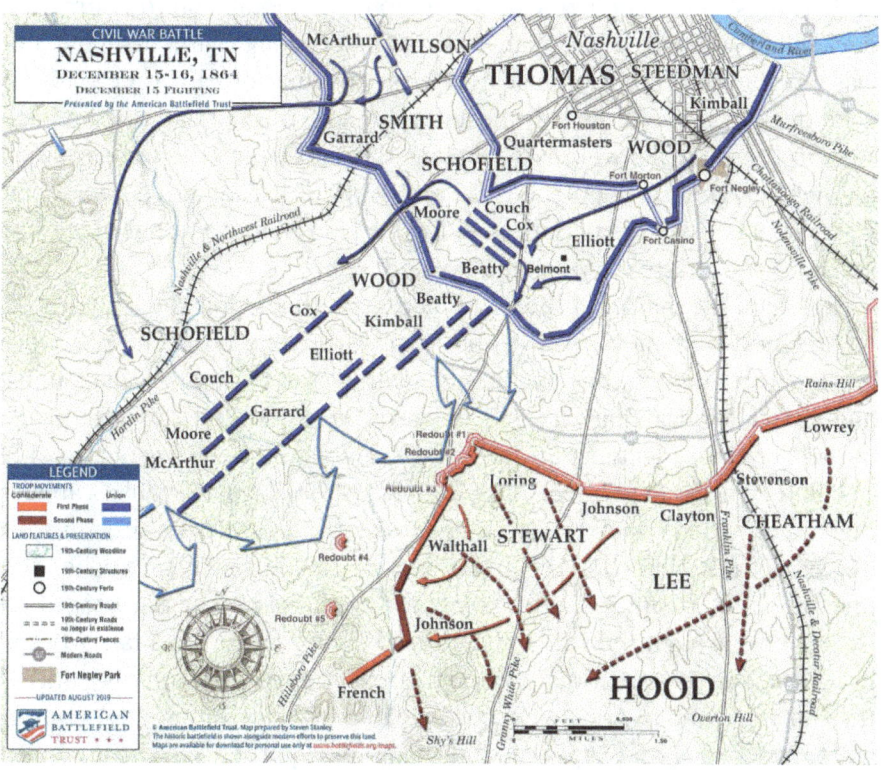

26-1: The Battle of Nashville

The U.S. Army Hospital Steamer D.A. *January* waited at the Cumberland River landing after the Battle of Nashville to transport wounded soldiers to either Louisville or Nashville.

The D.A. *January* (FIG. 502) was a side-wheel steamer which served as a floating hospital. Outfitted by the Western Sanitary Commission, in the fall of 1862, it was designed to be the best in patient care. On the hurricane deck (FIG. 503), the roof of the boat, was the Texas, on top of that the pilothouse. The staterooms were taken out and the whole cabin deck converted into one spacious ward (FIG. 504). Long windows were placed on all sides of this ward, attached by strong butts along the center of the ward. About the center of this deck, on one side, was a nurses' dining-room, a bath-room, and water-closet, and on the other a special diet kitchen, bath and wash-room, and water-closet. Away aft there was on one side a drug-shop and steward's room, on the opposite side a linen-room, in the center an operating-room. Drinking-water throughout the ward was drawn from faucets placed at convenient distances. The bath-rooms were supplied with water from a large tank on the hurricane deck, filled with water by steam-power. The drinking-water arrangement was a refrigerator on a large scale. Pipes ran from the tank on the hurricane deck into two large ice-chests in the hold of the boat, one on each side. In these chests were large worms through which the water passed and was carried through the different wards, furnishing iced water, or water cool enough for all purposes. By this plan a large amount of ice was saved, as the chests were seldom opened.

Between the main and the boiler decks, on the middle deck (FIG. 505), where the wood-racks used to be, two wards, one on each side, were arranged, containing thirty beds each, with water-closets, wash-troughs, and faucet for drinking-water. The wards were low, but the bulk heading was composed almost entirely of windows, so that plenty of air could circulate. On the lower deck (FIG. 506) there was a comfortable ward for one hundred beds, water-closets, and wash-troughs; a large kitchen connected with the wards on the upper decks by a dumb-waiter; a bakery on one side, a blacksmith shop, carpenter shop, and commissary room on the other. Through the whole length of the main ward ran a fan, worked by steam from below (it made about ninety revolutions a minute), and as the transom windows opened just above it, at the sides, it created a pleasant current of air and kept out all flies and mosquitoes. This boat carried from April 1862, to August 1865, altogether twenty-three thousand seven hundred and thirty-eight patients. It regularly visited the cities along the Mississippi and Ohio rivers.

History: Built in Cincinnati, Ohio, 1856; side-wheel steamboat, 450 tons; 225 ft. long; 34 ft. beam; 65 ft. extreme width; two high-pressure engines, 22-inch cylinders, 7 ft. stroke; additional donkey engine connecting with a steam-pump for fire protection. Purchased by U.S. Government, spring, 1862; after alterations it made first trip in April 1862, to Pittsburg Landing, arriving in middle of Battle of Shiloh, loaded with large supply of hospital stores and ended up transporting a total of 2,133 wounded soldiers, from Pittsburgh landing, on six separate trips.

According to Dr. John Vance Lauderdale book *The Wounded River*, from April until September 1862, the steamer carried more than 3,000 patients from battles, involving both sides of the conflict, traversing over 8,000 miles on the Mississippi, Ohio and Tennessee rivers.

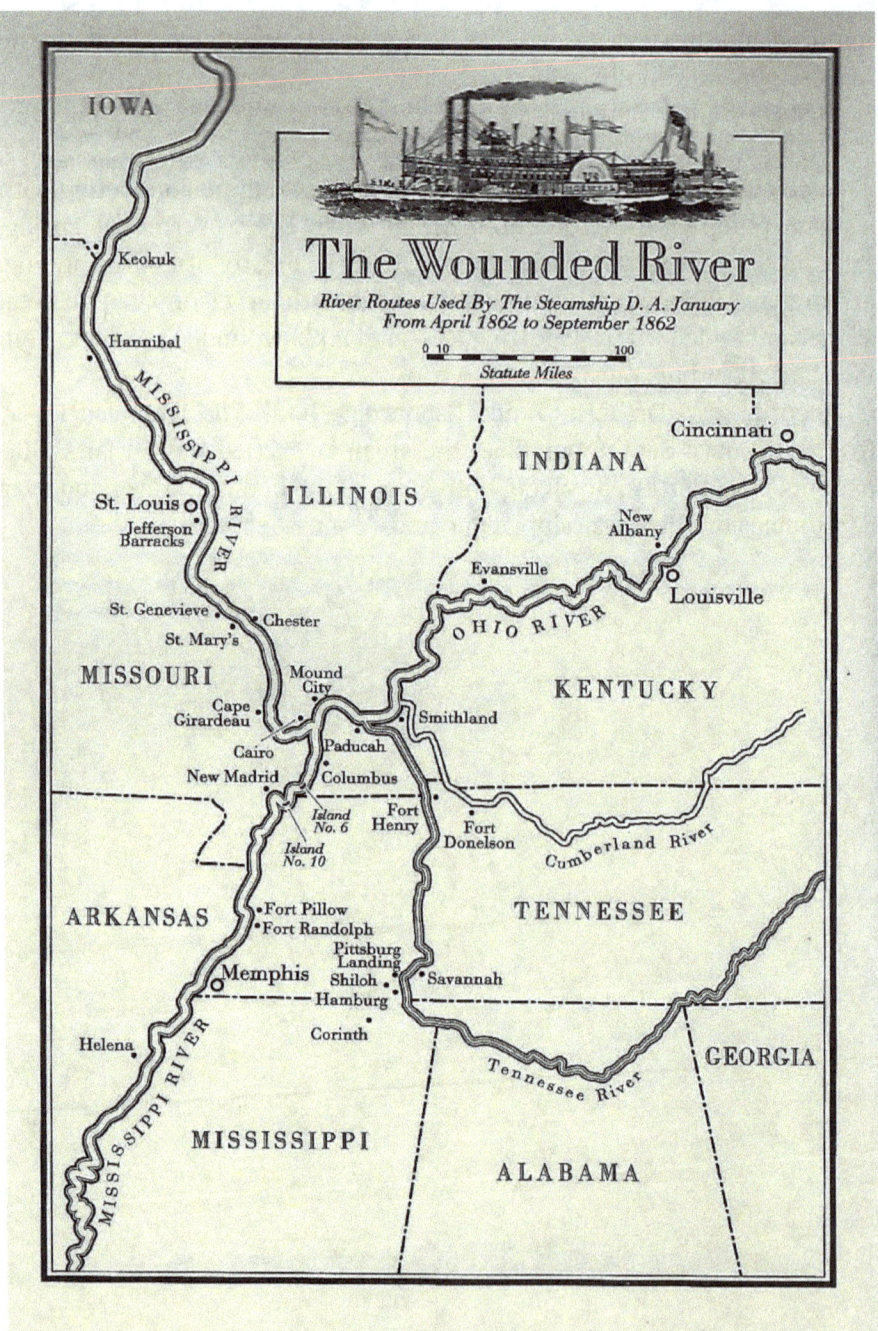

26-2: River Routes made by the Steamer D.A. January from April-September 1862

The D.A. January (26-3) was a side-wheel steamer which served as a floating hospital. Outfitted by the Western Sanitary Commission, in the fall of 1862, it was designed to be the best in patient care. During March, April, May, June 1863, this ship laid near Milliken's Bend, Louisiana, serving as floating hospital for armies under General Grant.

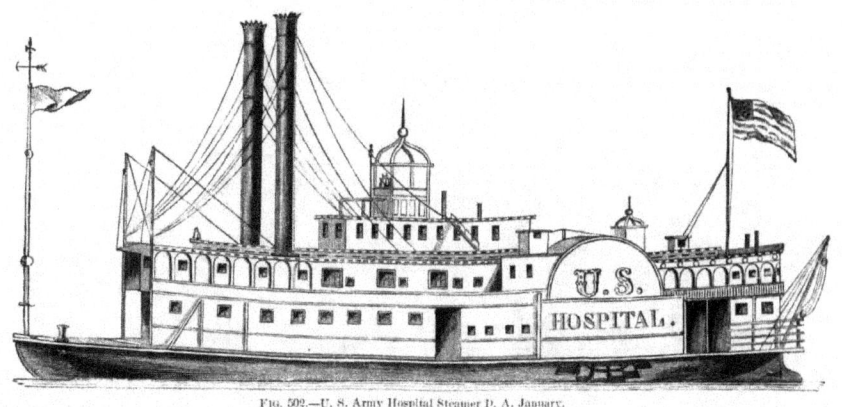

26-3: Hospital Ship D. A. *January*

On the upper hurricane deck (26-4), the roof of the boat, was the Texas, on top of that the pilothouse. The staterooms were taken out and the whole cabin deck converted into one spacious ward (26-5). Long windows were placed on all sides of this ward, attached by strong butts along the center of the ward. About the center of this deck, on one side, was a nurses' dining-room, a bath-room, and water-closet, and on the other a special diet kitchen, bath and wash-room, and water-closet. Away aft there was on one side a drug-shop and steward's room, on the opposite side a linen-room, in the center an operating-room. Drinking-water throughout the ward was drawn from faucets placed at convenient distances. The bath-rooms were supplied with water from a large tank on the hurricane deck, filled with water by steam-power. The drinking-water arrangement was a refrigerator on a large scale. Pipes ran from the tank on the hurricane deck into two large ice-chests in the hold of the boat, one on each side. In these chests were large worms through which the water passed and was carried through the different wards, furnishing iced water, or water cool enough for all purposes. By this plan a large amount of ice was saved, as the chests were seldom opened.

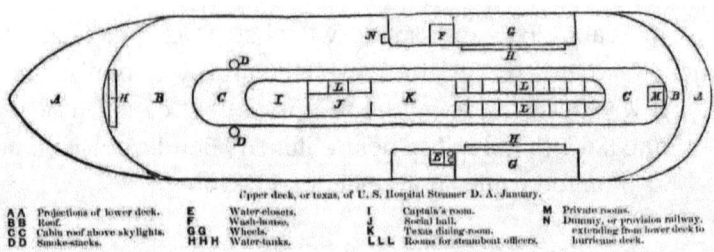

26-4: D.A. *January* upper deck

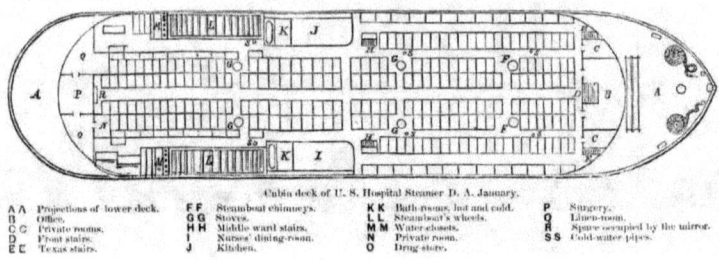

26-5: D.A. *January* cabin deck

Between the main and the boiler decks, on the middle deck (26-6), where the wood-racks used to be, two wards, one on each side, were arranged, containing thirty beds each, with water-closets, wash-troughs, and faucet for drinking-water. The wards were low, but the bulk heading was composed almost entirely of windows, so that plenty of air could circulate.

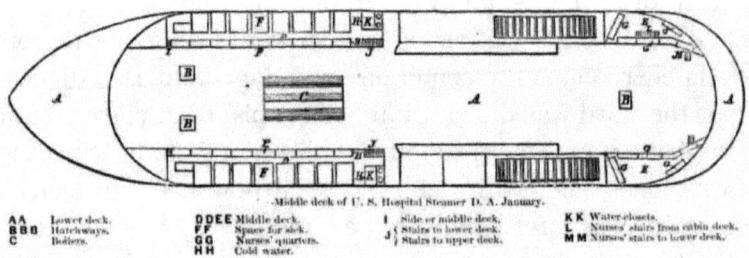

26-6: D.A. *January* middle deck

On the lower deck (26-7) there was a comfortable ward for one hundred beds, water-closets, and wash-troughs; a large kitchen connected with the wards on the upper decks by a dumb-waiter; a bakery on one side, a blacksmith shop, carpenter shop, and commissary room on the other. Through the whole length of the main ward ran a fan, worked by steam from below (it made about ninety revolutions a minute), and as the transom windows opened just above it, at the sides, it created a pleasant current of air and kept out all flies and mosquitoes. This boat carried from April 1862, to August 1865, altogether twenty-three thousand seven hundred and thirty-eight patients. It regularly visited the cities along the Mississippi and Ohio rivers.

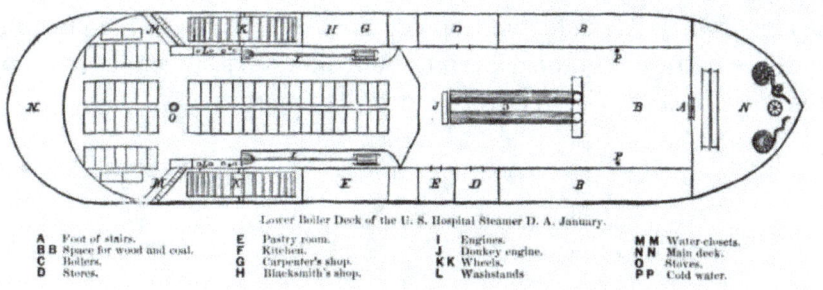

26-7: D.A. *January* lower deck

The D.A. *January* was used on Ohio and Mississippi Rivers from 1862 - 1865. By August 1865, it had carried a total of 23,738 patients.

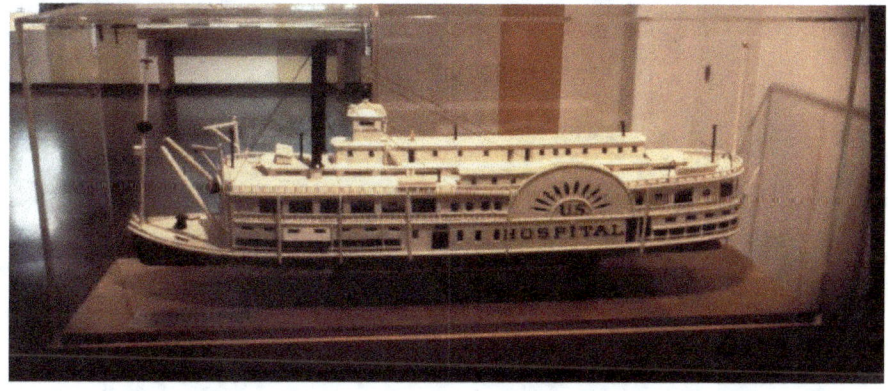

26-8: Model of the D.A. *January* at National Museum of Health and Medicine in Silver Spring, Maryland. It was originally constructed for Centennial Exposition 1876 at Philadelphia.

CHAPTER 27
The Campaign of the Carolinas

The Campaign of the Carolinas (January 1 - April 26, 1865), also known as the Carolinas Campaign, was the final campaign conducted by the Union Army against the Confederate Army in the Western Theater. On January 1, Union Major General William T. Sherman advanced north from Savannah, Georgia, through the Carolinas, with the intention of linking up with Union forces in Virginia. The defeat of Confederate General Joseph E. Johnston's army at the Battle of Bentonville, and its unconditional surrender to Union forces on April 26, 1865, effectively ended the American Civil War.

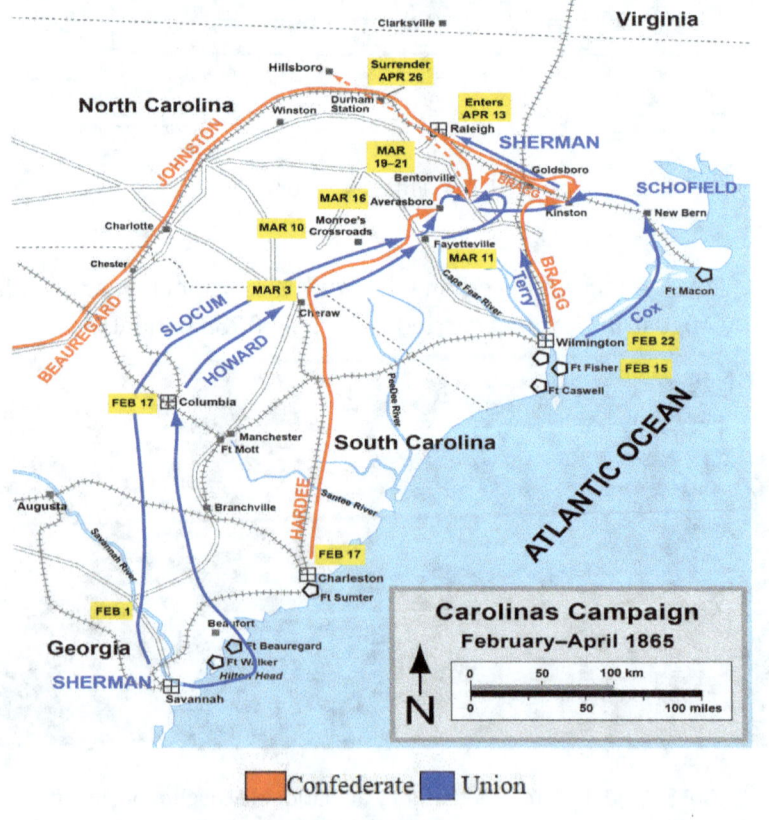

27-1: Campaign of the Carolinas

The hospital ship *Spaulding* was dispatched to meet the army when Sherman presented Savannah to Lincoln as a Christmas present in December of 1864. Coastal steamers fitted as hospital ships, evacuated the wounded from depot hospitals in Savannah to hospitals in the New York, Alexandria and Philadelphia. As Sherman's army moved north, additional hospitals were established in Beaufort, Charleston and Hilton Head South Carolina.

In support of Sherman's Carolinas Campaign, the hospital ship *General J.K. Barnes* embarked 2,137 sick and wounded Union soldiers from Savannah, Georgia, Hilton Head, Beaufort, South Carolina and Wilmington, New Bern and Morehead City, North Carolina to the DeCamp General Hospital on Davids' Island, New York.

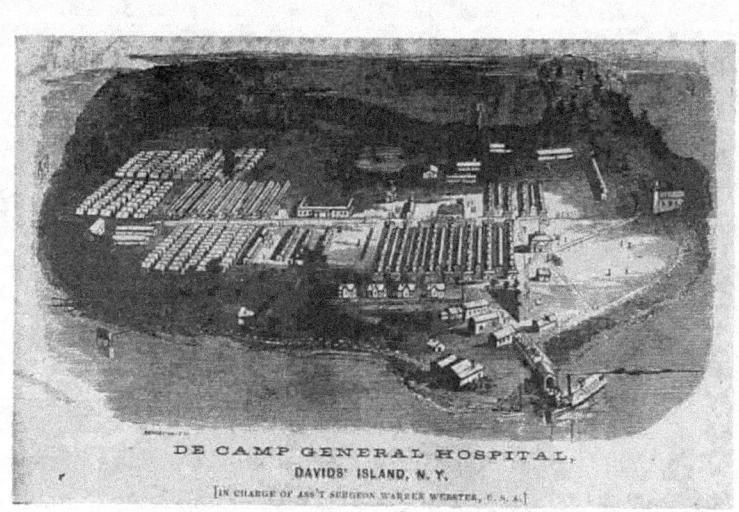

Plate No. 2. Woodcut of DeCamp General Hospital, Davids Island, N. Y., in 1863.

27-2: DeCamp General Hospital

In addition, the *J.K. Barnes* delivered wounded soldiers to the McDougall General Hospital in Fort Schuyler, New York (320), Grant General Hospital in Willet's Point, New York (119) and general hospitals located in Washington, D.C. (385) and Alexandria, Virginia (375).

Wounded soldiers brought to Alexandria, Virginia by railroad and vessel crowded the available hospitals and temporary medical facilities in and around the town. Many of the largest buildings in town, including The Lyceum, were confiscated for use as hospitals.

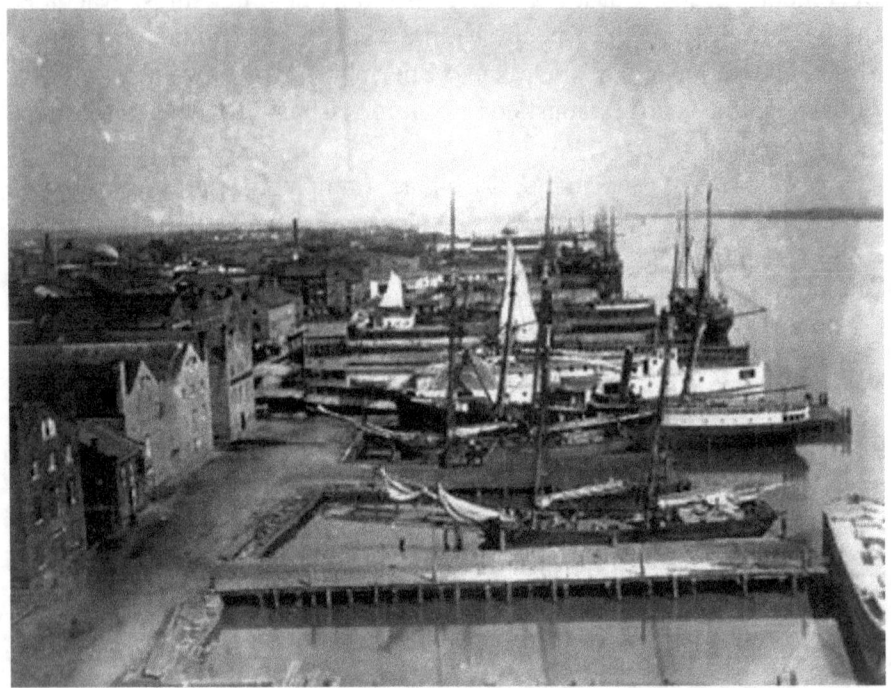

27-3: View of the harbor at Alexandria during the time of the Civil War which received hospital ships such as the J.K Barnes.

The *J.K. Barnes*, named after Surgeon General Joseph K. Barnes, was one of 14 coastal steamships outfitted as a hospital ship to convey the wounded from field hospitals in the south along the Atlantic coast to hospitals in Alexandria, Philadelphia, and New York City. In November 1864, it was outfitted to carry 449 patients, under the supervision of naval architect Charles Hemje and Assistant Surgeon Alexander Hoff U.S. Army, who had experience managing the evacuation of wounded soldiers along the Mississippi River during the western campaigns of 1862 and 1863.

and around the town. Many of the largest buildings in town, including The Lyceum, were confiscated for use as hospitals.

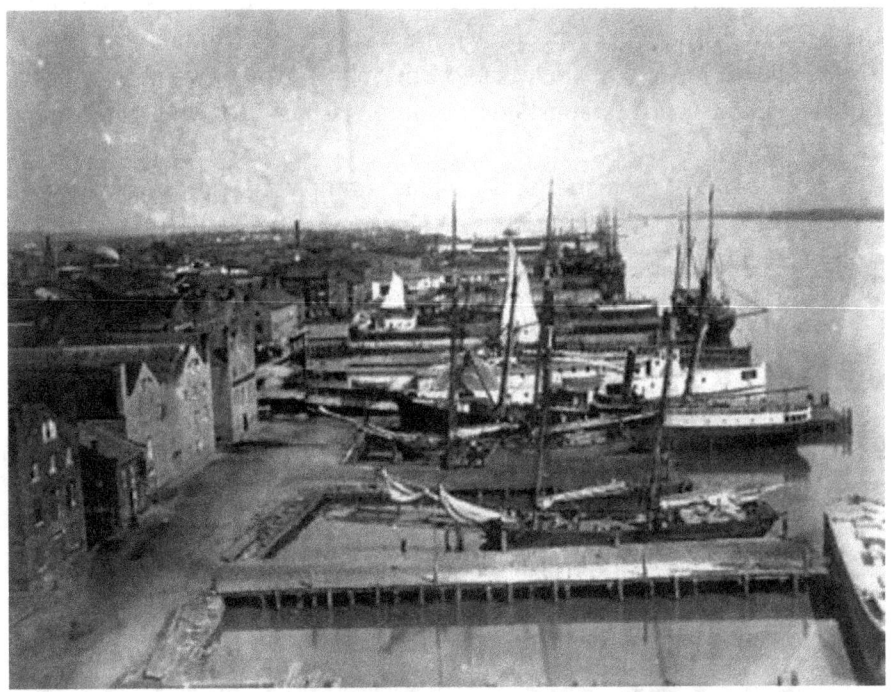

27-3: View of the harbor at Alexandria during the time of the Civil War which received hospital ships such as the J.K Barnes.

The *J.K. Barnes*, named after Surgeon General Joseph K. Barnes, was one of 14 coastal steamships outfitted as a hospital ship to convey the wounded from field hospitals in the south along the Atlantic coast to hospitals in Alexandria, Philadelphia, and New York City. In November 1864, it was outfitted to carry 449 patients, under the supervision of naval architect Charles Hemje and Assistant Surgeon Alexander Hoff U.S. Army, who had experience managing the evacuation of wounded soldiers along the Mississippi River during the western campaigns of 1862 and 1863.

The hospital ship *Spaulding* was dispatched to meet the army when Sherman presented Savannah to Lincoln as a Christmas present in December of 1864. Coastal steamers fitted as hospital ships, evacuated the wounded from depot hospitals in Savannah to hospitals in the New York, Alexandria and Philadelphia. As Sherman's army moved north, additional hospitals were established in Beaufort, Charleston and Hilton Head South Carolina.

In support of Sherman's Carolinas Campaign, the hospital ship *General J.K. Barnes* embarked 2,137 sick and wounded Union soldiers from Savannah, Georgia, Hilton Head, Beaufort, South Carolina and Wilmington, New Bern and Morehead City, North Carolina to the DeCamp General Hospital on Davids' Island, New York.

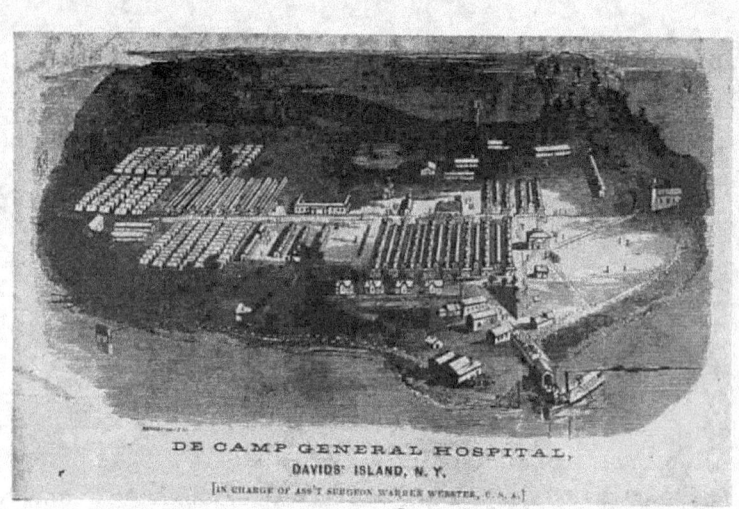

Plate No. 2. Woodcut of DeCamp General Hospital, Davids Island, N. Y., in 1863.

27-2: DeCamp General Hospital

In addition, the *J.K. Barnes* delivered wounded soldiers to the McDougall General Hospital in Fort Schuyler, New York (320), Grant General Hospital in Willet's Point, New York (119) and general hospitals located in Washington, D.C. (385) and Alexandria, Virginia (375).

Wounded soldiers brought to Alexandria, Virginia by railroad and vessel crowded the available hospitals and temporary medical facilities in

The Campaign of the Carolinas | 203

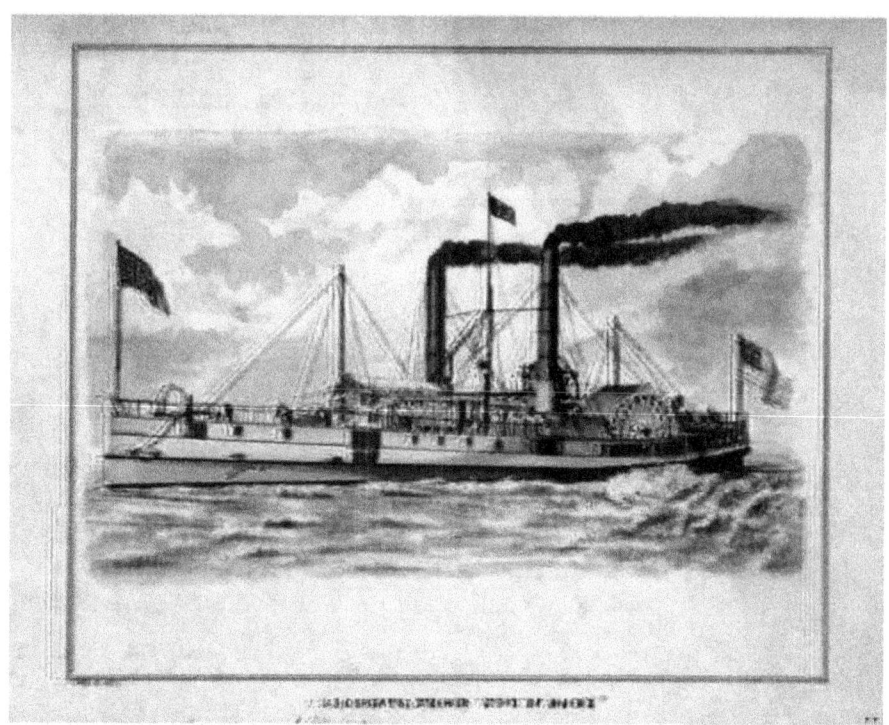

2662, HOSPITAL SHIP GENERAL J.K. BARNES.

27-4: Hospital Ship *J.K. Barnes*

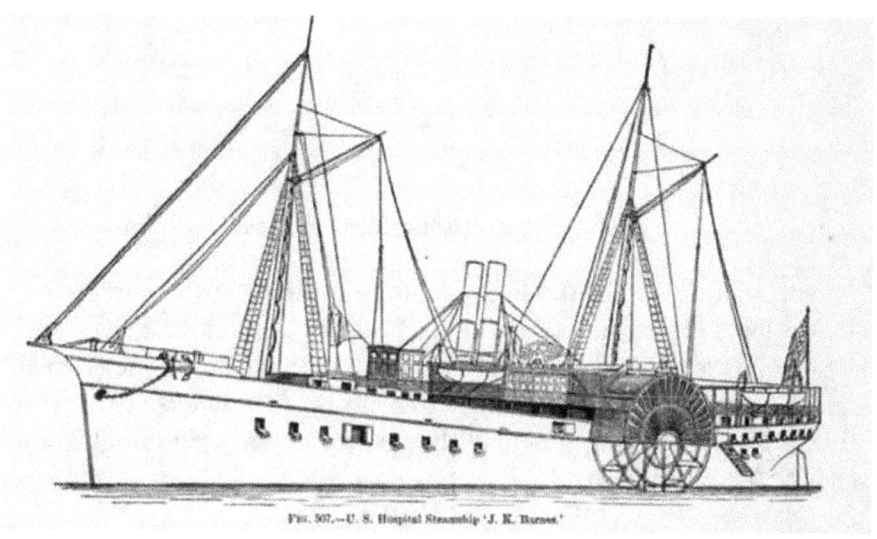

27-5: Hospital Ship *J.K. Barnes*

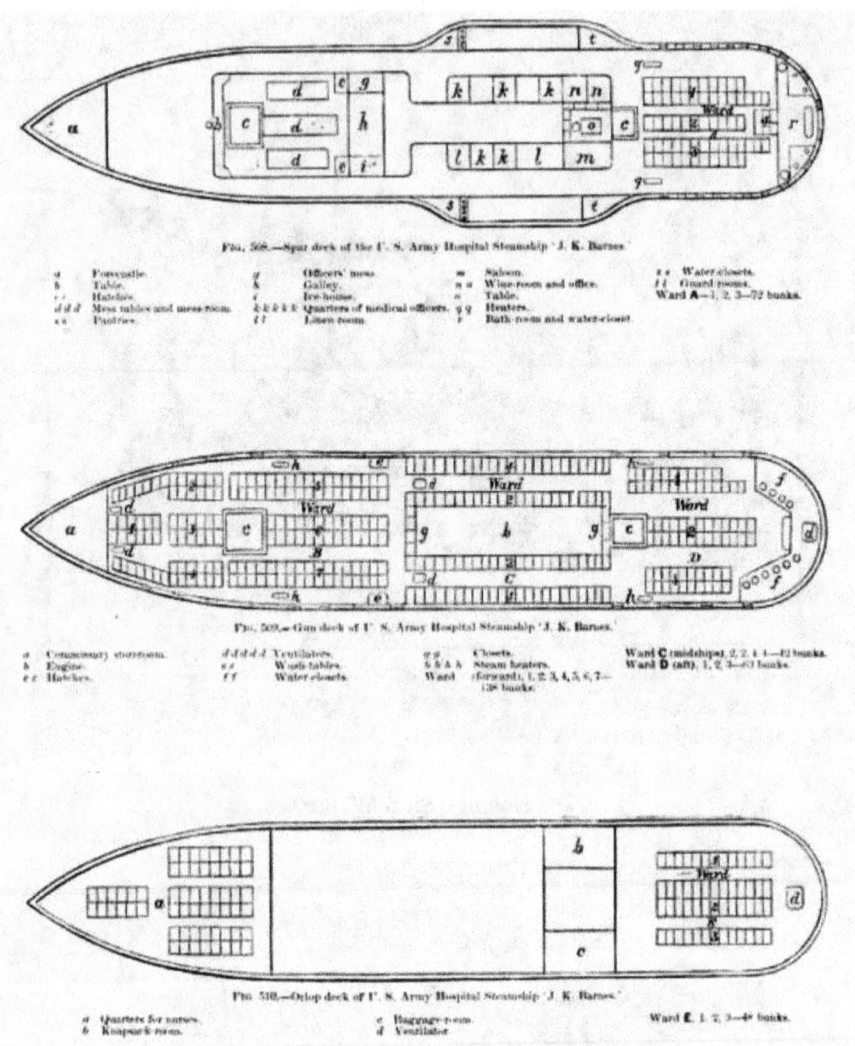

27-6: Decks of Hospital Ship *J.K. Barnes*

Representing one of the best adapted hospital ships of the period, a model of the *J.K. Barnes* was produced for the Centennial Exposition of 1876 in Philadelphia. It was used to show the public an ideal example of contemporary coastal steamships transporting wounded soldiers; the model of the *J.K. Barnes* detailed the intricacies involved in outfitting a vessel as a hospital ship.

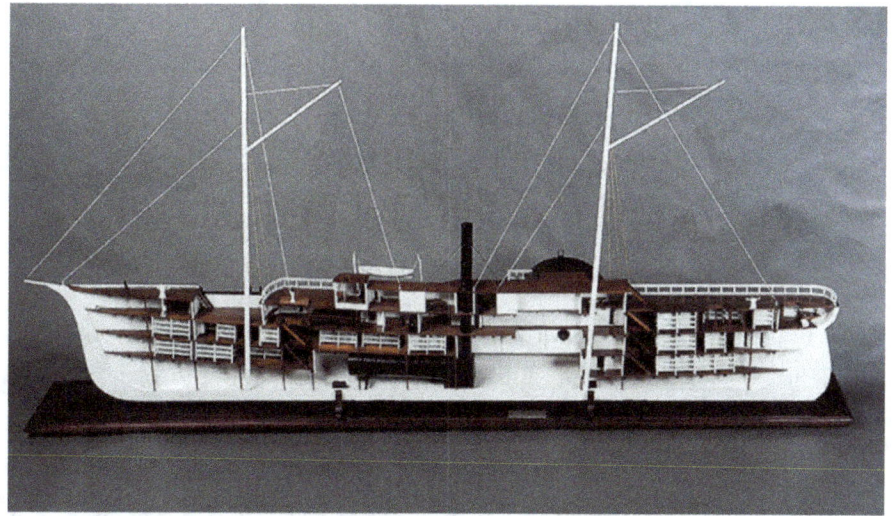

27-7: Model of the *J.K. Barnes* was produced for the Centennial Exposition of 1876 in Philadelphia.

The 8-foot model of the *J.K. Barnes* was identical to its 223-foot original, having been crafted by the same architect, Hemje. The cutaway model shows everything, from its exterior details like the paddlewheel, to the lower deck hospital wards and engine room. The model also displays the upper deck bathrooms, general cafeteria and galley, and the main deck officer's cafeteria, cabin, bathrooms, and wheelhouse.

Another hospital ship most likely involved in the evacuation of wounded Union soldier, especially from Savannah, Georgia, was the *Nelly Baker* embarking from Hilton Head.

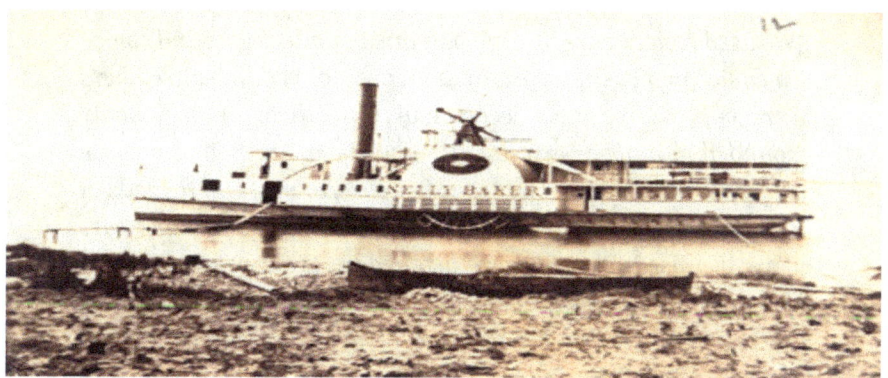

27-8: Hospital Ship *Nelly Baker*

CHAPTER 28
The South's Approach to Transporting its Wounded by Rail

"A Report on a Plan for Transporting Wounded Soldiers by Railway in Time of War, By George Alexander Otis, 1875"

"Few published statements have appeared respecting the transportation of sick and wounded in the Confederate armies."

"Preston Moore, Surgeon General of the Confederate Army, states in August 1875: "Freight and open box cars were used to transport our wounded from the field to the hospitals. In the beginning of the war these cars were bedded with straw or leaves, whichever was most convenient. It was soon found that this bedding became so foul as to be very unpleasant. This plan was therefore discontinued, and the wounded were placed on blankets, when they could be had, spread on the floors of the cars. Stretchers were not used. * * Passenger cars were not used for severely wounded patients, the freight and open box cars being preferred. The Confederates had no regular system of hospital trains. As far as possible this idea was carried out, but oftentimes the exigencies of the service forbade its regular adoption."

Dr. Hunter McGuire, Medical Director of General T. J. Jackson's Corps, remarks, upon the same date:

> "We used freight cars in transporting wounded men, and sometimes sick men, using straw or dry leaves for bedding. Stretchers were very scarce, and occasionally an officer or very badly wounded man was permitted to take one away. Sometimes we suspended one of them by ropes fastened to posts on the side of the car. We had few ropes, and no rubber rings. Passenger cars were also used. Planks were fastened on the tops of the backs of the seats; these slats were covered with beds, upon which the patients were laid. I remember only one regular hospital train, running from Guinea's Station [about twelve miles from

Fredericksburg] to Richmond. It was made up partly of freight and passenger cars arranged as above represented."

Dr. Howell L. Thomas, who was stationed in or about Richmond during the war, relates the following facts on the subject:

"Freight cars and flats were very generally used for the transportation of the wounded. The floors of these cars were usually covered with dry leaves or straw, as the locality best afforded; and in the absence of those, the best use was made of blankets, and other spreads, for relieving the hardness of the floors. Stretchers were not much in vogue, especially at the latter part of the war, when their scarcity prevented much resort to them. All sorts of intended comforts were improvised by attendants from the limited means at command. There were no ropes or rubber rings in stock. Passenger cars were converted to the use of recumbent passengers by laying temporary supports of boards upon the seats or the backs thereof, converting them into bunks, and making them hold two patients. Stretchers were used in such cases when they could be had. There were regular hospital trains once a day or oftener, from post hospitals to the field. They were in charge of regular medical officers with their aids, who were furnished with such supplies as would serve in emergencies. These trains were composed of freight and passenger cars, and the patients were quartered in one or the other according to their condition. Many of the passenger cars, if my recollection serves me, were bunked up (2 or 3 tiers) on the sides. But, except for emergencies, this close order was not resorted to."

Historians have generally shortchanged the South's hospital trains, but the Confederacy certainly ran them on a regular basis and from an early date. However, these hospital trains never achieved the sophistication and operationally contained status of those found in the North. In October 1861 the Virginia Central Railroad built two ambulance cars designed to hold 44 casualties each, distributed over 22 single and 11 double berths.

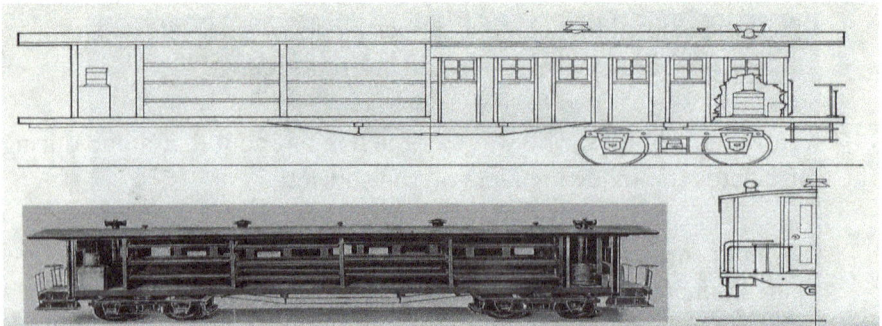

28-1: Hospital car with berths

The Virginia Central Railroad was an early railroad in the Commonwealth of Virginia that operated between 1850 and 1868 from Richmond westward for 206 miles (332 km) to Covington. During the war, the Virginia Central was a key element in Virginia's vast rail network, the most extensive in the South. The line remained largely in Confederate hands throughout the war and was essential to the rapid movement of troops and supplies, especially between Richmond and the Shenandoah Valley.

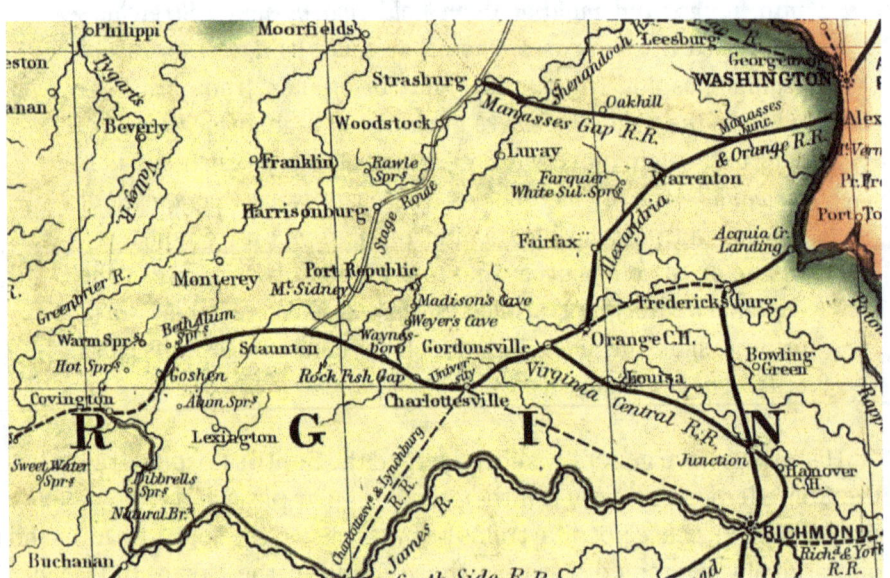

28-2: Virginia Central Railroad